Understanding Health

Understanding Health

Health

An Introduction to the Holistic Approach

EDGAR N. JACKSON

SCM PRESS
London

TRINITY PRESS INTERNATIONAL
Philadelphia

First published 1989

SCM Press
26–30 Tottenham Road
London N1 4BZ

Trinity Press International
3725 Chestnut Street
Philadelphia, Pa. 19104

British Library Cataloguing in Publication Data
Jackson, Edgar N. (Edgar Newman)
  Understanding health.
  1. Holistic medicine
  I. Title
  613

  ISBN 0–334–02401–3

Library of Congress Cataloging-in-Publication Data
Jackson, Edgar Newman.
   Understanding health: an introduction to the holistic approach /
  Edgar N. Jackson.
     p.   cm.
  Bibliography: p.
  ISBN 0–334–02401–3
  1. Health.   2. Holistic medicine.   I.Title.
  BA776.5.J25   1989   89–4494
  613—dc20

Typeset at The Spartan Press Ltd, Lymington, Hants
and printed in Great Britain by
Richard Clay Ltd, Bungay, Suffolk

To Pen and Marshall
friends indeed

Contents

Introduction

When I began this book five years or more ago, what may be called 'mini-systems' occupied the health care field and caused suspicion, jealousy, and friction. This has rapidly changed since what is now called 'psychosomatic' medicine has been widely adopted even by much of the medical profession itself. The revolution has occurred, but it needs to be better understood and further implemented. And it is even more important that the integration occur in the person being treated than even in the specialist who is administering the treatment. And this whether he or she be medical doctor, minister of religion, psychologist, or therapist.

Fractional systems, or what I call 'mini-systems', are not confined, of course, to the practice of medicine and the work of the ordained minister. They are found also in science, politics, economics, and almost every area of modern life. And since all of these callings contribute to the truly healthy individual and the healthy society, we need to take all of them into account in our analysis of holistic medicine. We will call this a 'systems' approach, but it is wider and more inclusive than the usual connotations of the modern-day usage of the term systems. The unifying factor is spiritual. And this spirit needs to become so widespread that it is compulsive. It appears as a sense of responsibility which is internalized and then made active.

A factor has been introduced into the consideration of health care that has not been an active concern for centuries. It has been so much a matter of discussion in the last few years that the subject has been overworked. Yet it is invasive and cannot be escaped. The AIDS epidemic has catapulted the personal behaviour of the human race into the centre of the picture. As never before in modern ways of thinking the moral responsibility of people of all races and creeds has been highlighted. The ways of interpreting this concern varies from the fundamentalist judgment to the curse of the libertine but all feel the threat of the ways of living that play fast and loose with sex and careless human relations.

People are thinking of what they do and the meanings of their attitudes in new ways. The medical profession is exploring new ways of controlling behaviour to relieve it of some of its implications. And yet more people of serious vein are thinking of sickness and sin with renewed interest and are modifying their ways of living with quiet determination not to be found wanting. To say the least a new sense of responsibility comes into life in ways that are changing patterns of acting and thinking. Those who have been thinking of a different means of modifying personal behaviour in relation to health may seize the opportunity to see life and the lifting of it in a vastly different way. Instead of the self-centred philosophy of a few years ago the 'me' generation may feel impelled to think in terms of a 'we' generation where we gladly give up some of our arrogance for an understanding of how we may learn a new way of dwelling together in righteousness and peace.

In the pages that follow we try to look positively at how we may meet the challenge of the present and future with a deeper understanding of what it means to be a person in this age. Without wallowing in recrimination we want to see clearly what the present situation is and how we can be part of the solution rather than part of the problem. It will take clear thinking and a willingness to abandon old ways of doing things. 'New occasions teach new duties and time makes ancient good uncouth.' This is our mood and this our determination. What will happen can only be found by our determined effort.

The germ 'spiritual healing' stimulates various emotional responses and mental judgments. It can conjure up the picture of a television evangelist urging people to touch their sets and feel healing power. It can cause people to think of unexplained remissions of painful symptoms. It can suggest the healing of wounded spirits so that bodies may be set free from the physical evidence of functional distress. It can even suggest unscrupulous manipulators of people's fear of pain and disease. Or it may imply the quiet intercession of Quakers on the one hand and the extremist behaviour of snake-wielding mesmerists on the other.

In these pages we will be thinking of the healing power at work in life in quite a different way. We will be exploring co-operative ventures of members of the healing team who share responsibility for true wholeness of being. In this context we will recognize the resources of those who work within the scientific disciplines as well as those who seek to discipline the non-material resources of life so that they may more fully participate in the processes of overcoming illness and preventing disease.

During many years of working with sick people and the professional persons who care for them, I have seen evidence of the significant non-physical and non-medical resources that work towards true wholeness of being. I have seen wise and unwise activities by both medical and non-medical people. I have tried to evaluate objectively the roles that may be assumed by various members of the healing team as they work with mutual respect and shared appreciation of their special skills.

My respect for the discipline and knowledge of medically trained persons was developed through three years of study at the Postgraduate Center for Psychotherapy in New York where the faculty and the student body were primarily physicians. Also during two years I served as visiting professor on the paramedical faculty of the Mayo Hospital at the

University of Minnesota and for ten years was consultant and special lecturer on crisis psychology at the Walter Reed Hospital and Medical School. These contacts have enabled me to see some of the biomedical process from the inside.

My appreciation of the role of the disciplined religious member of the healing team has grown from many years service as a parish pastor and a chaplain in mental, special and general hospitals. Thousands of hospital and sick room visits through the years have given me an appreciation of the possibilities for co-operation that may exist among those who share a common concern for the sick and a mutual respect for each other's contribution to the treating of those who are ill.

Both the religious person and biomedical person tend to operate from a mini-system of thought and feeling to which they give their major loyalty. So a mood of defensiveness emerges when the mini-system is challenged. Such defensiveness often stands in the way of larger emotional as well as intellectual understandings. The need is for a holistic approach that can bring together the best insight and the most commanding loyalties of all parties.

For several years I worked on a committee of the National Council of Churches which was assigned the task of clarifying a basic philosophy for modern medical practice. Made up of about equal numbers of physicians, phychiatrists and philosophers we struggled for years in the marshes of the mini-systems and seldom caught even a glimpse of the foothills of a maxi-system. Perhaps in these pages we may move a bit closer to a view of what a maxi-system might look like.

Because this book is about real people and shared human relationships, the illustrations used are authentic. Out of respect for professional confidence and personal dignity the details are modified to protect identity without destroying the dynamic quality of the human experience.

1

From Fractions to Wholes

Nearly twenty-five centuries ago Plato recognized the integrative nature of holistic medicine in saying that the great error of the physician is in failing to recognize the interdependence of the soul and the body. The trouble with Hellenistic physicians, he continued, is that they are ignorant of the whole, which ought to be studied at the same time as the particular complaint.

Compare this with the conventional biomedical statement of approach, which even today asserts that health is the absence of disease. Sanitary conditions ought to be considered, but social, psychological and spiritual dimensions are rarely involved in ordinary interventions. But things have changed. We are in the midst of a health care revolution. Old ways are being abandoned and new attitudes, assumptions and actions are taking their place. Some areas are as strident as a politician arguing for health care insurance while others are as silent as the mood of the meditator.

The revolution has so many facets that we may not be aware of its implications for our lives. We need to take time to sort out the various evidences of change so that we may assess their meaning. Unless we look carefully at what is happening we may find that some of the effects of change are producing the opposite of what we seek. For years the physician has been the authority on health matters but now there are many and conflicting authorities as psychologists, nutritionists, hypnotists, physical culturists and faith healers make their claims.

Often personal authority takes the place of medical authority. As never before people are taking an active interest in doing the things they think will benefit their health. With strong conviction that provides the emotional incentive for their action they are adopting types of behaviour believing that what they do is good for them. Often their conviction is more apt to be supported by strenuous action than by rational examination and sound research. This combination of strong feelings and strenuous action without careful research can lead to unfortunate results. This is especially true if the person has some emotional instability to start with.

It is also true that people steeped in research on illness and disease who are preoccupied with its limited findings tend to eliminate large segments of human experience related to healthful activities. So the biomedical establishment has given minimal attention to nutrition, meditation, spiritual intervention and the non-material considerations related to illness and health. For instance, in one medical encyclopaedia I consulted the only reference to health involved health insurance and the topical index skips blithely from harelip to heartburn.[1] Here conviction and research tend to ignore the possibilities of personal responsibility for the prevention of illness and disease.

These conflicting attitudes tend to produce a polarization between those in the traditional biomedical mode of practice and those who seek a more holistic approach to health. The former works through chemical agents, surgery and electronic medicine. The latter are more concerned with the natural processes for maintaining or restoring homeostasis and intropsychic balance. This polarization can be unfortunate for the solutions to most problems tend to be inclusive rather than exclusive.

My feeling is that the problems of illness and health in our world are so monumental that they call for the sharing of all insight and practical resources. A 'both-and' approach rather than an 'either-or' stance is essential if we are to march into the twenty-first century with a full utilization of every resource for understanding and remedying the ills of humankind.

In order to move beyond this polarization with its built-in tendency towards self-destruction we need the perspective of a relatively new discipline reflected in the systems view of persons. It may be wise at this point to look at the processes of polarization as they occur in human experience. How does the revolt against old philosophies of healing manifest itself? How do the biomedical disciplines tend to restrain personal responsibility for more healthful living? Let us look at some real people who illustrate this quiet and yet insistent revolt going on in our culture.

One woman I know is so concerned about nutrition that she travels many miles each week to buy her family's food supply in a health food store where she pays more for less. She firmly believes that vegetables grown in a natural way, that is without chemical fertilizers and sprays, are better for her and her family than foods that have chemical additives and other ingredients that may impair the body chemistry of those she cares for.

Another person of my acquaintance rises early each morning and jogs several miles. To hear him talk you would think that this exercise was a source of salvation. He says it gives him time to think. In fact he claims that he is nearer God with his deep breathing than anywhere else on earth. He claims that he improves his heart action, his lung function and his general body tone. He has become a jogging missionary and actively works to get his friends to share this early morning activity with him.

A physician friend has installed a whirlpool bath in his yard where he can spend an hour each day in utter relaxation as the hot water swirls about him stimulating healthful circulation of blood at the same time that it takes the tension out of his muscles. In this way he avoids the taxing rigors of strenuous exercise and provides what he thinks is a wiser form of health

3

care. He is sure that the psychological and spiritual effects are worth the time also. He finds further benefits by adding a social dimension to his experience. He invites others to share his pool and the rich soul conversation that takes place has none of the side effects of muscle strain or skeletal damage.

Yet another person has discovered a method of meditation that she claims has transformed her life as it improves her health. Each morning and evening she sets aside thirty minutes of inviolable time to engage in self-emptying. She focusses on the most meaningless symbol she can imagine with strenuous mental discipline until she has reduced the content of her consciousness to as near nothing as possible. In this state of utter nothingness she feels the pressures of life are reduced and her blood pressure stabilized at a desirable level. She claims she worries less and lives a more placid and pleasant existence.

A 'successful' business man says he has found the true secret of health. Years ago he discovered that when he was concerned about other people he was miserable. He decided to put himself first. In business he learned the skill of firing people without remorse or discomfort. He was promoted as efficient. He became skilled in riding roughshod over other people and their feelings. He said that if it came to ulcers he would rather give them than get them. While he might not have many real friends there are lots of people trying to stay on the good side of him and that seems to satisfy him. He has power over them. The money that came with success made it possible for him to buy the good things in life and that too made him feel good. Why worry about others? Live for yourself and you'll stay healthy.

At a fiftieth college class reunion a man in his early seventies was constantly being congratulated because he looked so well, so young and so prosperous. His hair was plentiful with just a touch of grey. He stood erect and dressed with stylish good taste. When he was asked how he explained the difference

4

between his condition and that of most of his classmates, he said it was all due to three things. In the first place he had chosen the right set of parents to give him desirable genes. Secondly, he knew how to quit and get out of the rat race, so he retired at fifty-five. Then he was free to work as much or as little as he chose, being a consultant. Lastly, when in college he had taken a course in philosophy which explored 'The Golden Mean'. This was an approach to life temperate in all things. He had adopted its philosophy and it seemed to have worked well for him.

Here we have a half-dozen practical programmes for achieving health, each a mini-system. Quite obviously health is not so much a definition as it is a way of life, a pursuit of wholeness of being. If we are to talk intelligently about health and our responsibility for it, we will want to stay close to the practical and realistic. So as we look at the personal patterns reflected in the six paragraphs above we will want to evaluate them as to their effectiveness. What happened to these people?

Nutrition is important for life, for though we are always more than what we eat, what we ingest has a bearing on our health. I can think of three persons who made a fetish of a stringent diet, denying themselves meat, or eating mostly rice, or limiting their food intake to raw vegetables and fruit. Each of these persons had read a popular book or articles advocating the advantages of a particular diet and decided it was for them. With stern discipline they adhered to their chosen diet. One was hospitalized for glandular malfunction and submitted to surgery for correction. Another became obsessed with rice and had to cope with a nervous disorder that grew with her obsessive behaviour. The third experienced a major disruption of her social life because she put food first and the benefits of a pleasant and healthy social life second. The importance of nutrition, which cannot be denied, may most effectively be considered in relation to a variety of other things that need to be thought about to keep life in a healthful balance.

No one would deny the importance of reasonable exercise. Speaking recently at a seminar on public health, a professor of orthopaedic surgery at Dartmouth Medical School said that as long as jogging is as popular an activity as it now is the need for orthopaedic specialists will increase and the incidence of injuries to knees and ankles will become more common. This is not because jogging is unwise in and of itself, but rather that the excessive activity at weekends on improper road surfaces damages the soft body tissues. While it would be unfortunate to discourage wise exercise, it seems important to relate exercise to age, body condition and environmental situations. As with nutrition, a programme of exercise usually produces best results when the needs of the whole person are taken into consideration. Exercise at its best is a means to an end rather than an end in itself.

My physician friend with the hot whirlpool bath is wise to provide for a reasonable amount of relaxation in his life. Stress causes organic breakdown and relief from stress is essential. But, like everything else, there is need for discipline even in relaxing. Given a choice between hard work and relaxation there are few who would opt for hard work. My friend the physician has become so enthusiastic about his jacuzzi that he can't wait to get home from his office, spends increased time in the comforting waters, and has reduced a normal programme of exercise to the diminishing point as creeping indolence claims more and more of his life. It takes no great insight to perceive that too much relaxation may be as hazardous as too little. Relaxation as a way of life can atrophy creativity. Relaxation as a resource is surely desirable, but as an end in itself, it can disturb the healthful balance of creative action and wise response.

The interest in meditation has been with us long enough to make it possible to assess some of its results. Those who use methods of meditation that are designed to empty the thought content of consciousness and fill it instead with the ultimate of

6

meaninglessness tend to find that at first they feel relieved of stress and experience physical benefits. But when the process is continued, the beneficial results are reduced. Then in order to continue the benefits, the programme is stepped up with more time and effort. This can lead to dissociation and a break with reality. Most normal people drop out of the programme when it ceases to be beneficial. The more tenacious are apt to persist until they are in need of psychological help to bring reality back into focus.

Life can be enriched by wise and creative meditation, but it shows a lack of respect for the magnificent gift of consciousness to destroy its primary function which is to give meaning and direction to life. We determine whether our meditation is creative or destructive. We would seek to fill consciousness with the richest meaning we can discover. We would focus consciousness on the highest good we can know. Meditation is beneficial health-wise and other-wise when it is a quest for meaning worthy of the gift of life. It is important to understand how meditation is used, for it too is a means to an end and not an end in itself.[2]

The business man who would rather give ulcers than get them is a member of a large group in our culture. Courses in aggressive behaviour are popular. Here you can learn to take advantage of others before they can take advantage of you. It sounds good on the surface. A strong offence is the best defence. It can even be fostered as national policy. But what is this model really saying? It is glorifying power and manipulation in place of understanding and compassion. There is a type of mental or emotional disorder that is called psychopathy or sociopathy. People who suffer this disorder are deprived of the capacity to relate kindly to other people. They learn instead to make their way in life by gaining power over others so they can manipulate them. Some people have this way of life thrust upon them by cruel circumstances in early childhood. It seems unfortunate that others would try to

7

develop these same traits as a way to achieve business success.

Any indications of healthfulness that come by creating callousness in human relations are bought at a high price and may not have long term benefits. If a person wants to make personality changes it is important to know that the whole person changes in the process. To buy success in business as the price of failure in the more significant aspects of life is a poor bargain. Here again we see that wise approaches to health require a more complete and perceptive understanding of the nature of true health of being. To adopt a way of life that avoids ulcers in return for a change of personality that impoverishes the human dimensions of being is cheating the self indeed. A philosophy of life needs to be big enough to support all of life, not just a small fraction of it.

The youthful seventy-year-old at the college reunion was smart enough to know that life has given qualities that we cannot change. We do not choose our parents, our height or colouring. We may choose our weight. We receive at birth a whole set of built-in traits that will stay with us for life. They will set some of the boundaries of life, but even our heredity is amenable to some modification depending on what we do with it. Proper exercise may give strength to a heart with an inherited weakness. Careful diet may help control an inherited digestive weakness. Maintaining control of life and daring to make changes when they may seem beneficial may modify a genetic weakness. Setting a pattern of temperance and wise moderation can mean that a person remains in control of life rather than having life exert an unreasonable control over him or her. Many of the so-called accidents of life may be more completely under our control than we realize. There are no external crises. There are only external events. The crises emerge from within as we process the events that are a part of our experience. We can work to stay in charge rather than drifting aimlessly in response to outside forces. Our coping skills will in the long run have a bearing on our health.

.

We have looked at half a dozen ways people use to assume responsibility for their health. Probably few people carry their health activities to extremes. Most of us would combine thoughts and actions relating to our health. To that extent we are already responding creatively to the revolutionary changes that are taking place in health care and the personal responsibility we assume for our own health. However, the time has come for more extensive and better organized ways of thinking about our philosophy of health and our responsible behaviour in relation to that philosophy. That is what we will try to do in this study.

We have seen that we have in our culture many ways of acting out our feelings about health. We also have ways of saturating our language and our awareness with concepts of illness and disease. Through popular magazines and television programmes we are made aware of the technical language used to dramatically describe illness. If you ask a friend recently hospitalized how he or she is doing, the response is apt to be a detailed description of symptoms, treatment modalities and physical responses that will be laden with the technical language of the health care professionals.

Our verbal behaviour can subtly influence our thinking as our language develops with a disproportionate emphasis on illness and disease. Just take the matter of words we have available in our language to describe wellness or euphoric states of being. We can probably count on one hand the words that apply to health – well, sound, feeling good. We are impoverished in verbal equipment for articulating our thoughts about good health. Perhaps that is why people act out health interests in bizarre ways, for the alternatives of talking about them are so limited.

Inversely our language is abundantly weighted toward words that describe morbid states of mind and body. On a shelf of dictionaries in front of me I have a medical book that lists thousands of words that are the technical equipment of the physician for talking about illness and disease. Next to it is a psychiatric dictionary with eight hundred pages of words that describe unhealthy states of mind and spirit.

If we are going to develop a wise and useful way of talking and thinking about our total health we will have to learn some skills to define what we are talking about. This effort is not new. Efforts have been made to this end over long periods of time but without much impact on our perception. Let us look at some of these efforts and see how they may serve our purpose.

Leonard Cottrell, for many years a social psychologist with the Russell Sage Foundation, speaks of health as 'the progressive maximizing – within organic limits – of the ability of the organism to exercise all of its physiological functions and to achieve its maximum of sensory acuity, strength, energy, co-ordination, dexterity, endurance, recuperative power, and immunity'.[3] Here the emphasis is on physical function.

The Constitution of the World Health Organization defines health as a 'state of complete physical, mental and social well-being, and not merely the absence of disease or infirmity'. Here we have a recognition of the role of body, mind and society in the creating of a healthful state of being.

In a recent article in the Hastings Center Report these observations were made: 'A sense of well-being is the essential feature of the healthy individual. The precondition for health is the integration of the physiological, psychological, and spiritual dimensions of the individual.'[4] Here spiritual considerations enter the picture.

The contrast between the last two definitions tends to set the philosophical basis for the polarization that now exists and may indicate the areas of exploration that must be approached as a prerequisite for setting new standards for understanding the nature of health and the important human needs that must be confronted.

What do we see in this brief exploration? The difference

between biomedical approaches and holistic concepts are a different view of health, one positive and the other negative. This leads to a different understanding of disease. The medical view is that disease is a 'deviation from the norms of measurable biological variables' while holistic perspectives see disease as 'more than a simple pathological agent'. Rather it is 'an indicator of disharmony between the individual and his/her environment or a disintegration of the essential dimensions of the individual'.[5]

Healing for the medical tradition involves co-operation with the physician so that the disease can be conquered, usually by consumable products or services such as drugs, treatments, operations or hospitalizations. With the holistic concept there is an added dimension. The relation to the doctor provides more than pills. The patient-physician relationship assumes a more active role in the patient to the end that life is reintegrated and the physician works with the patient towards that end. The role of the patient is more passive with traditional medical practice and more active and creative with holistic approaches. The physician is obliged to relinquish some of the authority of traditional medicine in order to stimulate a more active role and greater responsibility on the part of the patient using the holistic model.

2

Spiritual Bases of the Meld

How does healing happen? Because all healing uses the resources of the healee, the variety of ways for it to happen are as numerous as the persons to whom it happens. It always happens as a process. The differences in the way it occurs may be in elapsed time or in the agencies employed in the process. Alexis Carrel watched lesions close before his eyes at Lourdes and said that in each instance the normal process was followed and the major difference observed was in the time it took.[1]

When a patient with inoperable calcium spurs in her neck was referred to me at Walter Reed Hospital where I am on the staff as a consultant in crisis psychology her neck was stiff and she appeared to be in pain. Following a period of counselling and prayer I placed one hand over the affected area of her neck and the other on her forehead and continued in prayer. The patient claimed an immediate reduction of pain and demonstrated an increased lateral movement of her head and neck. She also, without prior question, described a tingling sensation all over her body which she said was like the way she felt when the physician gave her an injection of calcium during her last pregnancy. It could be that the calcium spur had dissolved into her bloodstream. Because it is potentially dangerous to overload the bloodstream with calcium, cases of this kind should be treated with several short sessions rather than with one long one.

When a patient was referred to me by a clinic after an electrocardiogram that showed heart damage and dangerous levels of stress, I used an hour of counselling, ending with prayer and the laying of my hands on his shoulders. The patient claimed strange sensations in the cardiac region. I recommended that he return to his cardiologist for another examination with possibly another electrocardiogram. The second reading showed a different set of tracings. His physician said the second reading showed no heart damage. Also he could return to a cautious work schedule. Further he said he had better have a technician in to check his electrocardiograph for it seemed to be 'cutting up'.

Two PhD candidates on whose doctoral committee I was serving presented theses that explored the subjective and objective criteria that would be used to assess the validity of healing in response to prayerful intervention. Both showed statistically significant results as measured by independent observers. Also, laboratory animals show a significant response to the directed energy of consciousness by visible modification of behaviour in controlled tests. A psychologist and a psychiatrist by focussed consciousness modify the content of dreams under test conditions. A research psychiatrist at the Menninger clinic finds that a number of psychoanalysts queried have evidence of telepathic interaction with their patients. There seems to be a growing body of evidential material that affirms that there is a healing force that can be generated through predetermined and controlled forms of intervention. It is obvious that we do not know nearly as much as we would like to know about the healing force, but we know enough so that we cannot ignore it with impunity.

It is one thing to describe some situations where healing has occurred. It is quite a different thing to explain what has been observed and described. There are apparently two separate processes at work. One has to do with the organic drive towards health that is present in every living thing. This life force has been looked at with philosophized interest by George Santyana in his book *Skepticism and Animal Faith*.[2] This movement towards health is a constant process concommitant with life itself. It can be interfered with by other internal and external forces. Yet physicians in their practice of biomedical intervention always have a positive factor on their side with animal faith at work. Much illness may involve active interference with this life force by psychological and other factors that block the normal healthy response to life. Any force that can reduce or remove these blockages will tend to release the drive towards health. Reassurance, social or family support, a change in focus or a stimulus to the processes of consciousness may well prove to be a healing force for a person suffering from an imbalance of body chemistry or of disturbed emotions. The literature of psychosomatic research is replete with illustrations of this force at work.

The other process at work which cannot be ignored involves the role of the so-called healer. Some of the people who appear to have special endowments in aiding the healing process have been carefully studied. Dr Lawrence LeShan has made such a study and reports on the people who stimulate active responses in the lives of others.[3] These people have differing philosophies to explain what they do but all seem to share a common set of traits. As a group they tend to be warm, sensitive, loving people who approach others with utter selflessness. During the time when they are at work they appear to be in states of intense concentration which shows up in altered states of consciousness. Almost invariably they are people who work within the three levels of nonmaterial reality and seldom charge fees or accept payment for their services. Dr Robert Laidlaw, formerly chief of psychiatry at Roosevelt Hospital in New York, in research he conducted reports what he calls a healing force generated by so-called healers which is characterized by a deeply penetrating and intense form of heat.[4] He claims that these persons have a spiritually dedicated and outgoing nature and also appear to have a higher component of psychic endowment. This is characterized by telepathic ability and similar abilities in psychic diagnosis and clairvoyant ability. This fits the findings of George Devereaux, Research Director at the Menninger Clinic, Topeka, Kansas, and Shafica Karagula who in two separate studies found that psychically endowed physicians tend to have enhanced diagnostic abilities.[5]

LeShan in his extensive study of so-called healers and the healing process observes that, in the act of healing, the healer and healee create a new and valid existential relationship which produces significant changes in the healee. 'All psychic activity is undoubtedly accompanied by some biochemical change.' In this state the so-called healer moves into quite a different level of psychic activity. 'In this moment of intense knowing on the part of the healer it was valid and the healee was an integral and central part of the system . . .' 'Knowing this at some deep level of personality, the healee was thus in a different existential position . . . In a way, he was for a moment in what I might call "an ideal organic position". He was completely enfolded and inclosed in the cosmos with his "being", his "uniqueness", his "individuality" enhanced. Under these conditions there are sometimes positive biological changes.'[6]

Dr LeShan continues: 'The healer, particularly those with a Christian approach . . . view "wholeness" and "holiness" as having the same meaning . . .' 'Ambrose and Olga Worrall wrote, "In true prayer our thinking is an awareness that we are a part of the Divine Universe".'

Speaking personally, I have hesitated to use the term healer because it seems to be presumptive and inadequate as a description of how I see my role. I think of myself as primarily a facilitator of responses within the person being healed or as a transformer of the energies that are God's nature into personalized forms that are more accessible to him or her. I feel all healing is of God and that it would be close to sacrilegious to claim it for myself. I think of myself as a joiner of things that should be together but for some reason have come apart. I use

15

the inventive creative resource with which I am endowed to help make something new and valuable in the persons with whom I work.

For instance, a healthy finger could be seriously impaired by tying a piece of string around it so tightly that circulation of blood was cut off. The finger would turn blue and the blood would deteriorate causing the finger to rot away with gangrene. If someone intervened early in the process and made it possible for healthful circulation to be restored the finger would be healed. If on the other hand the intervention was delayed until the finger fell off, according to all we know about human anatomy it would be impossible to restore the rotted finger. This same analogy might be applied to a number of other human conditions. Impaired thought processes could affect body chemistry and could be changed by religious experience or psychotherapy. If left unmodified, the unwise use of thoughts and feelings could poison consciousness and illness or death could follow.

As I write a phone call interrupts and the substance of the call is relevant to the subject that now engages us. I am asked to co-operate with some physicians in preparing a documentary videotape for educational television concerning a cancer case with which I worked last year. It concerns a young couple in Colorado who had an experience of acute grief. Their baby-sitter and their two children were killed when their car stalled on tracks in front of an onrushing train. The sorrow of these young parents for the death of their only children was rejected by a family and community that felt the only way to meet tragedy was with a stiff upper lip. So the grief found detours for its expression. A robust and healthy farmer who had never known illness was desperately ill with cancer in a few months. I heard of the family's need when the father was on his 'death bed'. Medical intervention was no longer useful. No solid food had been ingested for two weeks. At best the grieving father was given a week to live. Because I had lost two children

16

through accidents I could resonate to their grief. I called them and talked briefly with both about my belief that there was life after tragedy. They had read some of my books and appeared ready for a change of focus for their lives. He began to sleep well, ate breakfast the next day, and soon was up and about. It was as if the string had been untied. Life forces began to be manifest. The last time I called them they were on a weekend trip to the mountains. While he works the tractor he still must be careful for where cancer-damaged bone tissue exists there is still need for care to avoid fracturing fragile parts. Now instead of death there is life. I see my role as one who facilitated a change in attitude that produced a whole series of other significant changes in co-operation with other skilled and concerned professionals. This apparent recovery from cancer seems to verify the healing power of a maxi-system where several forms of intervention occur to bring about changes in body, mind and spirit. While I feel this is a valid revelation of the power of God at work in life I do not believe that it should be considered miraculous or magical. I feel that natural laws of life and health can be implemented without assuming that the law and order of the universe is compromised or interfered with. As far as I am able I refuse to explain the phenomena of life by a retreat in mini-systems when there is a better basis for our understanding of these phenomena in a systems approach to ultimate reality.

The basic ingredients in a fruitful healing process include at least four elements: the person needing healing, the person or persons who seek to facilitate the process, the laws of nature within which both must work, and the power of God revealed through nature and the natural endowment of human beings who are made in the divine image. Henry Miller brings these four elements into focus when he writes: 'The great physicians have always spoken of Nature as being the great Healer. This is only partially true. Nature alone can do nothing. Nature can cure only when man recognizes his place in the world, which is not in Nature, as with the animal, but in the human kingdom, the link between the natural and the divine.'

When we try to consider the philosophical and theological ideas basic to the healing process we are not dealing with concepts as such as much as we are with dynamic forces at work in and through people. There are many instances of persons with inadequate conceptual frameworks who are able to produce significant phenomena that can be observed and verified. We are well aware of the fact that healing can occur in most remarkable ways. Recently a man who had been blind and deaf as the result of a motor accident several years back was struck by lightning. Immediately his sight and hearing were restored. To assume from this that all that is needed to restore sight to the blind and hearing to the deaf would be a powerful electric shock would be misleading. On other occasions people struck by lightning have been killed. Such phenomena have to be explored in the light of best insight. To organize a cult of the lightning struck would be to pursue a mini-system to a ridiculous conclusion. Almost as misleading would be the idea that healing can occur only in response to injected or ingested chemicals. The accumulated human experience, clinical, case-oriented or anecdotal, provides so much evidence of numerous healing resources that it would be unfortunate to try to attach to any self-limiting mini-system. Rather we would seek a framework that is adequate to hold all the truth we can discover. This calls for the use of a maxi-system that can bring together all of the insight we can discover in our most innovative exploration of human behaviour and cosmological processes. Why settle for the limited when the unlimited is available?

What is healing? How does it happen? Who are healers? How do they work? There are no simple or easy answers. To seek or to settle for small answers could well shut us off from the next and great steps to be taken in discovering the realities that exist through the wonders of healing, human and divine.

3

A Systems Approach

One thing is clear, however. The systems approach which combines emotion and intellect is the basis of a valid systems approach to health. And we should never make the mistake of thinking that faith without intellect is a durable solution of the problem.

To round out our analysis of the spiritual approach to health, therefore, let us consider the intellectual content, because it is this in too many cases that is missing today.

Our task, first of all, is to try to bring some order to our understanding of the human mind and the products of mental activity. It is difficult for us to conceive of the rapid development of knowledge in recent times. A historian of contemporary thought[1] says that the total of human knowledge acquired before the year 1800 was doubled by 1900, and that total was doubled again by 1950 and yet again by 1975. How can this explosion of the products of the human mind be explained? At least three things can be mentioned. Eighty per cent of the scientists that ever lived are alive and at work now. They have the most sophisticated tools that have ever been devised to aid the human brain. Computers can solve in a few minutes problems that might have taken a scientist a lifetime before the advent of electronic devices. Scientists and inventors are not apt to be working alone like Edison, but share national and international pools of research such as the Geophysical Year. All of these resources working together have made it possible to expand knowledge in a reservoir of scientific information, technological skills and psychological insight. Certainly some technique for organizing this complexity of research findings and technological skills is imperative or we will drown in it.

Research relating to the human brain and functioning of the mind is pivotal. If the computer is organized after the model of the human brain, it is important to understand the brain to understand and control the computer. The researches of Lord Adrian and Sir John Eccles have given us some guidance in trying to appreciate the wonders of the human brain.[2]

Lord Adrian points out that the brain has roughly ten thousand million specialized cells. These cells are long, thin and mobile so that under certain conditions they can interact with about twenty-five thousand other brain cells. The special condition is when the brain is engaged in strenuous activity such as concentration on a problem of mental arithmetic that may be just beyond the capacity of the person to solve. Under the stress of this form of activity the brain cells tend to contract thus producing a scalloped-like surface which projects molecules through the cell wall. This process generates minute charges of electricity which in times of intense mental activity would be multiplied many fold.

One begins to get some idea of the magnitude of this mental process if one tried to raise ten thousand million to the twenty-five thousandth power. A group of people interested in science were having a retreat at our farm home. One of the physicists was a computer programmer for the National Aero Space Agency. I asked him what ten thousand million to the twenty-five thousandth power was. I was met with incredulity. Why should I want to know such a number? In the first place there was no such number for it was inconceivable to think of it, and impossible to make a computer that could cope with such a number. When I persisted my friend took an hour's walk in the woods, a break from our spiritual life seminar. When he returned he said he had a rough guess as to what it might be, give or take a few thousand zeros. He said it would be something like a one with a hundred thousand zeros following, or about thirty-five pages of zeros. When I looked incomprehending, he smiled and said another way to put it was the equivalent of the total number of molecules in our solar system, sun, moon, planets and the free floating material in interstellar space. When he insisted in wanting to know why I sought such an impossible number, I admitted that this was the amount of potential mental activity in the human brain in any given second.

Lord Adrian creates a concept of the human mind that makes us stand in awe and wonder. The kind of activity he describes makes it imperative that we move away from reductionism that studies human potential by watching rats in a maze. Only a systems view of the human mind could begin to bring such magnitude into comprehensible range.

The potential impact of mental activity on problems of health is made explicit, for instance, when the second volume of *Medical Research*, published by the American Foundation says: 'The correlation of electrical and clinical mechanisms in nervous function is fundamental to understanding the influence – old among the physician's problems and newer in medical science – of psychological and neural factors in disease and recovery . . . A change at one point, in one molecule even, may reverberate throughout the entire system to initiate changes in seemingly unrelated organs and tissues. This concept, familiar in physics, is gaining validity in all fields of biology and medicine.'[3] The implications of this process can be gauged by the assessment that each brain cell has about three million molecules. The mind or consciousness as the great systematizer is constantly at work to bring order out of apparently incompatible elements of life and experience.

The consciousness, for instance, works to give a systems view to the way we experience space, time, and motion. We live with different types of space psychologically. There is intimate space which is reserved for those with whom we would share the deepest and most personal experiences of life.

There is personal space which is reserved for those who are entitled to that next level of relationship beyond intimacy. Then there is social space that is regulated by rules of courtesy but shared only as these rules permit. Much difficulty arises when people trespass the boundaries between the intimate and the personal, and the personal and the social. It is reflected in the use of language as well as in obeying the rules of the road when driving a car. We are not formally taught these boundaries but they persist in all of life through the regulating activity of consciousness at work.

Similarly the consciousness as a systems organizer makes it possible for us to live in three different time frames at once without being disoriented. We live quite comfortably in chronological, psychological and cosmological time. We regulate our daily activities by clocks and watches for it is chronological time that governs news broadcasts and train schedules. Psychological time moves rapidly at some times and drags painfully at others. When we are enjoying ourselves time races, but when we are sad or suffering it seems that the distressing experience will never end. Yet in the midst of chronological and psychological time there is also the awareness of cosmological time, the fourth dimension that is at work reminding us of something within our natures that is aware of the eternal dimension of our own beings. We can live comfortably with these three concepts of time for consciousness correlates what may seem otherwise incompatible.

This function of the systematizing consciousness is even more dramatic with motion. We are able to travel at several different speeds at once without being ruthlessly torn apart. We can be walking down the aisle of a jet airplane at two miles an hour while it is travelling at six hundred miles an hour in an atmosphere that is travelling around the earth at a thousand miles an hour on an earth that is spinning around the sun at thousands of miles an hour in a solar system swirling through space even faster in a galaxy that is in motion at a rate of thousands of miles a minute in an expanding universe with greater and immeasurable speeds. Yet instead of being fractured by this incompatability of speeds we are totally unaware of it for an automatically functioning systems process solves our motion problems before we are conscious of their existence. Fortunately human consciousness and the cosmic processes of gravitation and inertia of motion work well together without any need for us to understand them for them to be employed.

Human beings are natural systems for organizing experience even though it is complicated. 'Any system that does not owe its existence to conscious human planning and execution is a natural system – including man himself, and many of the multiperson systems in which he participates . . . The most remarkable organic self-maintenance system is the process known as "homeostasis".'[4]

Science is a consciously designed and systematically reductionist approach to life and experience that excludes phenomena on the basis of its acceptability from the point of view of a scientific method that is exclusive rather than inclusive. 'The validity of the ends and means of medicine and of the models of man that emerge from them is a "transmedical" matter – one not susceptible to the methods of medicine itself.'[5] This reductionist approach begins with education when a person is admitted to the scientific community by engaging in a process of conditioning consciousness. Years are spent in an intense discipline which seeks highly specialized knowledge at the expense of more generalized understanding of the universe and its functioning. In the process the mind is honed to an effective level of denial of that which does not fit the system, the method and the discipline. Instead of knowing more and more about more and more, which would lead to the Leonardo de Vinci type of mind, the process in reverse tends to dampen creativity and limit the cross-fertilization within the mind that could be possible when the mind is set free to respond to its truly amazing potential.

In the scientific practice of medicine the tendency has been to limit the approach to human experience by eliminating all that is not objective. 'Special tensions arise from their conflicting claims to universality – medicine divinizing the body and the particular, philosophy the intellect and the abstract.'[6] 'In its pursuit of objectivity, medical science has grown relatively insensitive to the less measurable qualities of human life.'[7] These self-imposed limitations need no longer impair the perspective of medical science. The systems view of life and the universe gives to science an opportunity to incorporate into its activities a larger spectrum of observation and research at the same time that it is stimulating a new level of creativity that can save it from the restraints on truth that have limited its vision in the past.

What are the areas of research and understanding that would have to be incorporated in a systems approach to health and control of disease? Past experience may help us with an answer. Originally physicists developed a systems view of the universe to resolve conflicts and bring together incompatible theories. For instance, does electricity flow through waves or streams of particles? The answer was found not in an either/or dichotomy but rather in a both/and resolution of conflict. The truth emerges from what appears to be conflict when we discover a framework large enough to accommodate it. A systems approach offers the larger framework. In health care it is not so much a matter of biomedical or holistic perceptions as something larger than either, a new way of looking at people and their health that can bring together a number of forms of understanding to create something more than any of the components. So we are seeking something larger than the sum of the parts for something new is created and new meaning emerges when the systems approach is employed.

In simple analogy, what does a systems view represent? A baseball game is something more than the eighteen players engaged in it. A sentence is something more than words and their individual meanings. A symphony is something more than the sum of its notes. These practical systems we readily recognize and accept. Here we do not find it necessary to confront the self-limiting demands of a reductionist scientific method. With considerations of health we can move beyond the fracturing preoccupation with mechanisms and parts and consider the whole person in all the aspects of personhood.

What would be essential to such a consideration? First, of course, would be the physical equipment that is the focal point of the person. Second would be the impact of heredity. Third would be the influence of environment. Fourth would be the dynamic self. Fifth would be the non-physical force field, psychic in nature that empowers a person from within. Let us look at these basic elements.

We have already considered the physical in some detail. We have referred to the body systems at work in producing homeostatis and the mechanical phenomena that use muscle and bone and nervous system to produce a living and moving human being. In this amazing complexity it all starts.

Heredity brings together the generalized impact of long periods of development of racial traits and archetypal formulations. It also brings into living form the specialized traits that make it possible for children to look like their parents. Physical weakness or strengths may come along with these individualized characteristics. It also tends to show up in forms of illness that appear to have racial roots. Some genetic structure apparently is predisposed to specific illnesses. Black people are subject to sickle cell anaemia. Jewish people seem to be the exclusive victims of Tay-Sachs and Neimann-Pick disease. Diseases of the blood like haemophilia tend to appear when large amounts of interrelationship occur as in royal families. To ignore such clearly evident connections between heredity and disease would be unacceptable. A holistic approach could not ignore genetic contributions to health or illness.

The consideration of environmental factors has two facets,

the outside and the inside. The boundary is set by the skin. The only way we have of knowing anything about the world around us is through the skin and its various areas of refinement. The eye is skin tissue that is sensitive to light. The ear contains the skin tissue that is responsive to sound waves. Specially sensitized skin tissue provides the olfactory sense, the sense of taste and the tactile response. The skin is a richly endowed part of our bodies, with something like two million glands. Each hair follicle has three minute glands that help to control the response of the body to the environment's temperature. When it is hot the pores open and the glands secrete a fluid that evaporates rapidly and provides cooling. In cold weather the glands contract and provide protection against the temperature that might damage a warm-blooded creature. The glands can act instantly to produce 'goose pimples' or blushing, often emotional responses.

Often we fail to appreciate the wonder of the skin as the boundary between the inner and outer worlds of experience. The skin is a major portion of the body – about seventeen square feet in area and weighing three or four pounds if we do not count the supporting tissue and up to twenty per cent of body weight if we do count it. It protects the inner being from intrusion for even a pinprick is instantly sealed off with inner fluids. A relatively small bubble, if injected into the bloodstream, could be fatal. Held securely within the skin is an environment quite similar to that from which life originally emerged, with trace elements of many minerals and the complex composition of the lymph and blood which constantly carries life support ingredients to every cell of the body. If these body fluids leak out because of injury it could be fatal.

A second part of the environment is the person. We may not think of it but we are an important part of our own climate. We govern the processes of intake that support life. We can inhale or ingest what is damaging and injurious to the health of our bodies. So it would be unwarranted to discount the significance of that part of the environment of which we are so important a part.

Accidents happen. The fact that ninety per cent of the accidents happen to ten per cent of the people makes us aware of the fact that carelessness or unconscious purposefulness of the accident-prone is an aspect of life that affects health and disease. Not only are there mechanical accidents in our industrial and technological culture, but there are what doctors refer to as cardiac accidents, cerebral accidents, circulatory accidents and cardiovascular accidents. As forms of meaningful behaviour, accidents are certainly an important part of our experience as we confront matters of physical injury and bodily impairment.

Similarly, the ageing process must be considered as a factor related to disease and illness. Wear and tear on cells and organs begins before birth and continues with an ever increasing tempo throughout life. Slow deterioration seems to be a law of life and the war of attrition waged by the forces of gravity shows itself in the sagging of body parts, the loss of muscle tone and mental agility. Any holistic assessment of the forces at work to lay waste life would have to take into account the impact of ageing with an eye to its final triumph.

Yet another factor that must be considered is the unique and dynamic quality of each individual. As a result of extensive research on the placebo response, Dr Jerome Frank gave the dictum that a physician should not prescribe a specific medication until the placebo[8] response has been established. The attitude of each patient may vary enough to warrant a careful assessment of the body chemistry of each individual for what might be indicated for one would not fit the needs of another. Perhaps we never appreciated how significant these differences might be until the use of drugs like penicillin established the fact that what might be beneficial for most could be poison for some persons.

The dynamic self needs to be taken into consideration

constantly for we are learning that the attitude of a person may have a significant bearing on the nature of the illness and the outcome of therapeutic intervention. Surgeons hesitate to operate on a person in a state of depression because they know that various body systems are working well below their optimum condition and they want everything going for them when they employ such drastic modes of patient care. Patients can make themselves ill by the way they manage thought and feeling. Attitudes can be so powerful that they can reverse the effects of specific medication. In the John Hopkins experiments with placebos it was established that patients suffering from nausea could be administered an emetic (a specific to induce vomiting) with the strong suggestion that it would settle their stomach, and with a significant number of the patients it did just that.[9]

The dynamic self is an amalgam of developmental factors, personality traits and circumstantial forces at work in the life of a person. The way a person has been trained and the coping skills that have been developed with previous experiences become an active ingredient in determining the dynamics of selfhood. A person who had much illness in childhood and learned to use the illness as a source of power over other people will be apt to revert to the use of illness as a tool in later life. This may explain some hypocondriasis. Similarly a person who has learned to manage illness well early in life may be able to reduce its impact on life with later experience. Researchers have found two types of personality in response to physical sensation; the enhancers and the reducers. The enhancers amplify sensation and feel pain more intensely while the reducers minimize painful sensations. Aspirin is said to temporarily change enhancers to reducers.

The ability to use the dynamic self creatively can be learned just as the opposite is a learned response achieved by the effort to learn adaptive skills. 'Both Freud's death instinct and Selye's diseases of adaptation may be identified with those automatic mechanisms of the organism, the primitive, elementary and instinctive mechanisms, which are phenomenologically extraneous to the conscious ego. Freud similarly indicated that the "ultimate cause of the death of all higher organisms" is that they die from products of "their" own metabolism.'[10] This internalized climate under the control of the individual could be reversed. If the dynamic self could produce the diseased condition in the first place it would logically follow that the same internal processes could move in the opposite direction and restore health. Clinical evidence appears to support this conclusion in some cases.[11]

That these inner conditions have a relationship to a social system is also clearly indicated by research. James Lynch of the Johns Hopkins Medical School, after compiling statistics for ten years in the university hospital, says that in the intensive care unit, the cardiac unit and the trauma unit the patients who have more human contact even when comatose have a better chance of survival than those who are abandoned. In a study of survivors in prison camps in the Pacific it was shown that 'twice the expected number died of cancer and three times the expected number in accidents'.[12]

However, our major interest is not so much what we can learn from the negative manifestations of the power within, but rather what we can do to develop a systems view of illness and disease that can make it possible for us to organize and develop the forces within that can be used to create healthful forms of self-image and produce homeostatic and intropsychic states that will foster health. This will bring into a systems view of health the ways through which coping skills can be developed in the person, how personality traits can be enhanced and circumstantial factors can be managed more creatively. Then instead of having a scientific perspective that can fracture and frustrate the healing force, we can bring together and organize all of the insight that is emerging from the biomedical and holistic developments so that we can personally and culturally benefit from both forms of research and experience.

Let us now look more closely at the power within that may become a major resource in developing responsibility for health and for a better understanding of the systems view of total wellness and holistic well-being.

4

Using Inner Resources

Emotional energy is a primary fact of life. Love can stimulate heroic action and dedication to a purpose. Hate can be generated to produce non-rational action. During war and political campaigns it is not unusual for emotional appeals to fear and prejudice to be mingled with urges towards primitive loyalties. A holistic approach to health would seek to organize, discipline and direct the emotions that can create healthfulness and reduce those feelings that interfere with the optimum functioning of the organic system. We have come to the place where we can look at the concepts of emotions and bodily changes. We are ready to look at consciousness as the great systems resource of life as it brings together and directs forms of energy which take apparently disparate aspects of reality and meld them into a working force that stimulates creativity as it reduces conflict. Then we may be in a position to see how the products of consciousness become a vital force in matters of illness and health.

The inventive-creative potential of the human brain is the most magnificent product of creation. It functions to integrate and activate complicated processes that are well beyond the capacities of existing computers. It is now important for us to see how the potential can be made actual in our search for as yet unrealized resources for health. How does our systems organizer, our consciousness, work for us to accomplish these goals of healthful living?

We live in a world of what appears to be conflicting realities such as those of biomedical perspectives on life and health and the spiritual concepts of life and health. But in terms of consciousness they are not conflicting realities, but only evidences of the misuse of the resources of consciousness. We live with numerous aspects of reality impinging on our consciousness. By giving excessive weight to one mini-system or another we can distort the nature of reality by seeing only a portion of it. So the mini-system of the biologist is apt to over emphasize the findings of biology. Similarly the mini-system of the anthropologist will focus consciousness on but a part of reality which is important for limited types of human activity. So the psychologist may be so focussed on human behaviour and its meaning that the person gets lost in a flood of impulses, inner conflicts and developmental influences. Even the language of specialists tends to become a barrier to communication as these tools of consciousness become more precise. Fewer people know the esoteric language of the specialist so the circle of those with whom we can communicate shrinks. So we need a systems approach to organize and develop the possibilities of the various mini-systems.

Consciousness appears to be the resource that can bring together creatively the findings of the mini-systems with their limited supporting data. Let us look at six significant realities that constantly have an impact on our living. Quite contrary in their basic data, they are complementary when melded by the creative impact of consciousness. There is material reality, physical reality and artificial reality, all of which are bound up with the practical data of life and the daily experiencing of it. They are the realities that are the basic stuff of biomedical perspectives.

There are three other realities that we encounter in daily life that are less assertive and demanding of our attention but they are nevertheless important for they give meaning and direction to the first three. They are extra-sensory reality, transcendent, transpersonal or spiritual reality, and finally what we might call a mythic reality. They all sound rather abstract so it is important for us to give some practical illustrations of what we mean by the way consciousness brings together apparently contradictory realities. Before we use a medical or health-related illustration let us use one that is in a completely different field for it may sharpen up for us the principle we would want to make vivid and alive.

The reality of the material is all about us. It is implicit in everyday living. We know a material typewriter, a material chair at a material desk. We know they are there because we are continually experiencing them as there. This is the way we live our lives as we adapt and adjust to the reality that material things thrust upon us. But this material reality is known only by our physical equipment, sensory in nature and developed by the long process of experiencing. So the reality of the physical is added to the reality of the material. But the typewriter is not an extension of the self for it has its own separate and intrinsic quality. It is a process of consciousness that lies behind the experiencing that brings typewriter and person together in a creative relationship. This knowing has another practical dimension, for a long process of education and indoctrination adds to the material and the physical. This added reality is culturally acquired. It is artificial in that it is made by a group process in which we are all deeply engaged. A typewriter means more to a trained stenographer than to an Australian aboriginal who has never seen one before. The difference would be the end result of an artificially acquired concept of use and meaning. While it would depend on the material and the physical it would employ something more that is added, actually another reality important to life. This third reality, dependent upon the other two, varies from culture to culture, as meanings and use are perceived. So much for the three physically or materialistically oriented realities.

The three non-material realities are a more subtle but yet constant part of our experience. We are constantly using methods for extending the acuity of our physical equipment, therefore in simplest form these are extra-sensory devices. We wear glasses to see better. We use hearing aids to hear better. We turn on lights to extend our vision. We turn up the sound on our television set to hear better. At another level of extra-sensory usage the scientist uses electron microscopes to see what would otherwise be invisible. The astronomer uses a telescope to see beyond the bounds of normal vision. The physicist uses a cyclotron to explore forms of energy that can never be brought into the range of the physical senses. Thus we live in a world where the extra sensory is essential to our way of life.

There are other ways of knowing that do not depend on the three materialistically oriented approaches to reality. Our value system is constantly directing our response to life. We know things we have not learned in the classroom. How does a mother know that an eight pound baby is worth more than an eight pound leg of lamb? How does a person know that some things are right and some wrong? What is the basic material of ethical systems and moral values? And what about the way we use what appears to be another sense to know things without any form of communication except what we call telepathy? The energy of consciousness seems to create a psychic force field which is constantly at work shaping our responses to things and people. With this form of perception we seem to be able to move in and out of space and time as if some part of our being were free of physical limits. We may try to deny this reality but it is difficult to do for it is constantly at work to modify and enrich our experience in life.[1]

This extra-sensory awareness is certainly built upon the physical, material and artificial forms of reality, but moves beyond them. Something in the brain produces an inventive-creative addenum to experience that defies the limits that the physical and material would thrust upon us.[2] This inventive-creative process adds to creation itself something that was not there before so that in our use of this dimension of reality we are participants in the wonder of creation. We verify the divine image in our being as we continue the work of creation through the use and discipline of that portion of our being that is created in God's image.

This naturally leads us to the fifth reality that moves beyond the merely extra-sensory. We discover that this creativity of spirit adds another dimension to the inventive-creative process. Employing memory we can close our eyes and move backwards in time. No one is quite sure of the full meaning of this endowment, but we are able to relive life, explore new insights in relation to old experience and look into the future. In its more practical form we have market analysts and weather forecasters. We also have rare and largely undeveloped resources for organizing the content of consciousness to prophesy with clear vision of cause and effect processes that have not yet occurred in our chronological time frame. Much of the Bible is made up of prophesy. Julian Jaynes, in his provocative study of consciousness, sums up his quest with some eloquent phrases that focus on this inventive-creative reality. He says: 'The problem of the nature and origin of all this invisible country of touchless rememberings and unshowable reveries, this introcosm that is more myself than anything I can find in any mirror', is a supreme creation.[3] Fortunately there may be for us more positive conclusions than those he developed from his long look at the nature and origin of this inventive-creative aspect of being.

This fifth reality permeates our total life. We cannot live as if we do not remember. The occasional disorientation of amnesia is a terrible affliction. We cannot act as if we are bound to the present. Rich association gives us our history, our language and our personality. It gives us our sensitivities, our problems and our creative solutions. In creating a systems approach large enough to cope with our mini-systems we run risks and must accept penalties. The capacity for memory brings privileges and responsibilities to the systems potential of human

35

consciousness that we cannot escape for in a basic sense we are it.

A sixth reality of non-material nature is an aggregate of the human experience which organizes ideas larger than the life of an individual into composites that we call myths. Usually we do not know that we are dealing with mythological structures until we analyse their meaning or someone else points out to us their significance. Eliade and Malinowski have served our generation well in showing us the meaning and power of great myths.[4] Joseph Campbell has given a classic expression to the great myths of history in his book *The Mythic Image*.[5] A myth is not a false construction but is usually a great truth that stretches the bounds of usual language and so has to be expressed in allegory or symbolic form.

The great institutions of human history are steeped in mythology. The Roman Catholic Church has accreted about itself a rich treasury of mythology that has nourished the souls of millions through many generations. The ancient Greeks created a mythology that has fertilized human thought for ages. Even a young country like America has produced a significant mythology that was revealed forcefully at the celebration of its two hundredth birthday. Abraham Lincoln, dead a little more than a century, has centred about his memory a rapidly growing storehouse of mythological material. Families tend to develop myths that are shared on those occasions when members of the family gather to recall the past. When I was initiated into an honorary musical fraternity its open service was centred about Orpheus and the myths that were attached to him as a pioneer in creating beautiful music. Everywhere we look we see the impact of these great ideas upon us.

Perhaps no one has defined more imaginatively the usefulness of our myths than Carl Jung. Through his ideas about the collective unconscious and archetypal formations that are at work in the depths of our consciousness he has made us aware of aspects of our mental life we could easily ignore. These myths at the core of being constantly mould our personalities, concepts and attitudes. We cannot easily approach the wonder of consciousness and its ability to bring together apparently conflicting realities if we ignore such influences as mythology that shapes science, the arts, religion and ideas of illness and health. Witness the symbols of intertwined snakes on doctor's cars.

We live comfortably with these six realities even though each is a representative of a mini-system that shares differing perspectives on what is ultimate. It is only when they are bound together by a larger systems view such as that provided by the integrative force of consciousness at work that the problem is resolved.

We can see it well in the arts. Music, for instance, brings the six realities together in a maxi-systems approach. I attended the finals of the World Piano Competition in Sydney, Australia. Twenty young musicians, the best of their nations, each played a Mozart piano concerto. As I listened I tried to understand the consciousness processes employed. The piano was the material, an important tool of the artist, but surely the music was not there. The pianist provided the physical action with muscles, keys, levers, hammers and string all working together to start air waves in motion. But the music was not there. The artificial reality was provided by the setting, the tradition, the training and the personal traits and disciplines of each individual performer. These three objective factors were essential to creating the music, but if there had not been conscious listeners there the major factor in its creation would have been missing. The wonder of the ear, the refined tissue of the skin, the engineering feat achieved by the three little bones that transferred an airwave through a liquid and a solid to a nerve centre where the inventive-creative process was stimulated, all were essential to the creating of the music. But no one knows how this essentially non-physical process is achieved.

The auditory cortex which is material performs a creative function that is non-physical in its end result. And as if this were not enough the extra-sensory process can be recalled by the carrying out of mnemonic recreation. Years away in time, thousands of miles away in space, the music can be clear and vivid as consciousness works to fulfil its creative potential. All I had studied of music, its history and its performance through many years, provided a mythic base that was larger than the composer, the performance or the recall of it. To limit or reduce any of the six realities would limit or prevent the full process of musical revelation.

Perhaps through the following illustrations we can move our focus from the theoretical and abstract to the personal and the health related interests that demand the centre of our attention.

Let us look at the specific health problem to see how the various realities are at work to affect physical well-being. Bob Aldrich was a well-known radio and TV personality, with strong audience appeal. He had a fine intelligence and an easy manner as he interviewed the great and near great. He was recognized by top officials of the network and was promoted repeatedly. When he was notified that he was going to be considered for the top national spot and was to be carefully scrutinized for a year with every videotape reviewed and every programme examined for any flaws, his easy-going manner changed to tenseness. He slept poorly and became quite a different person at home and in the studio. Within a few months he developed a virulent form of cancer and on the day he had been scheduled to take over the new national programme he died.

What had happened to Bob Aldrich? In terms of the six realities what might explain his illness and death? The material in his body was torn apart and the life of his body destroyed by abnormal tissue developments. Physically he experienced disorganization accompanied by pain and increased disability.

The artificial reality within which he lived revealed a conflict between a man of great ability and reasonable ambition and a frightened child who was so threatened by the possibility of failure that a civil war raged within between the person of competence and the person who feared failure. At this point the non-material aspects of his case exerted their influence. It would be difficult to isolate the powerful force of fear that chronically affected his glandular response and upset the immune factor that impaired homeostatis. His body became helpless in the face of the emotional assault this unwisely managed approach to his intense feeling had produced. His inner resources, his spiritual power, was effectively cancelled by his anxieties. The myths about cancer, culturally amplified, added to his other fears until he was easy prey to the destructive forces let loose in him. It was only after his death that I had a chance to read his daily journal and sense the paralysing fears that dominated his life. The extra-sensory force of his life had turned towards self-annihilation as the unconsciously selected alternative to the failure he feared. The information we have presented is minimal and so able to reveal only the major dynamic forces at work. However, they may be useful in showing how the power of negative thoughts and feelings can bring together the six realities to illustrate how the unconscious power of this purpose behind the disease was so intense that it thwarted the counselling process and every resource of medical intervention that was employed. The six realities can be used to destroy life as well as to preserve it.

In the case of Elinor Olsen quite a different course was evident. She experienced acute abdominal pain and exploratory surgery showed metasticized malignant tissue in colon, liver and other visceral organs. With no effort to remove the neoplastic tissue she was sown up and chemotherapy was instituted, though the prognosis was not good and she was given a six month life expectancy. She had heard of holistic approaches to cancer. A crisis psychologist was called in and intensive psychotherapy employed in close co-operation with the oncologist and radiologist. An indepth exploration was made of emotional states that might be acted out viscerally such as repressed anger, hatred, fear and anxiety. A deep reservoir of these repressed feelings that had accumulated through life and never been openly confronted was explored. Hours were spent in pouring out agonizing hatred and resentment against family members. Often this recital of repressed feelings of hatred and frustration was accompanied by convulsive weeping. After a short period of counselling there was a marked relief of emotional stress. Active effort was made to restore right relationships. Coping skills were slowly and carefully developed. As insight was gained it was put to use through support group activity. New strength was found in a new self-image and new disciplines of meditation and prayer. The inner being was purified and creative reading was used to enrich the content of consciousness. Spiritual retreats were used to deepen the effectiveness of the mind's life. From these experiences a new person emerged, able to manage destructive emotions, organize the emotional life more wisely so that it supplemented other modes of medical intervention. Elinor became an active partner with all those who used professional skills to aid her recovery. She developed inner strength. Learning a new way of life has been a major achievement of her life and her physicians claim she has modified their perspectives.

The material body of Elinor Olsen cried out for understanding and there were those who combined their insight to interpret the body's metaphor. She responded physically and went through the processes of cultural shock that comes with facing advanced cancer. But she did something about it by engaging the three non-material realities and these powerful forces changed her life. She says that she no longer fears death but has learned so much from her painful experience that it is the most important thing in her life. She has found a new self and actively engaged the extra-sensory and spiritual resources that are important for her life. She has faced the old and destructive myths about disease and has plugged into a whole set of new myths, insights and feelings that have made her a different person, one she likes far more.

How we approach reality does make a difference. How we use our capacities of consciousness to organize and meld the various forces of life is a major concern of holistic health care. Let us move further to see how the resources can be developed.

5

Self Organizing Self

How can the self work upon the self? This has been a basic question of psychotherapy for a long time. It has been one of the prime concerns of religion in every culture. It has been the source of strenuous activity, sometimes cruel and futile and at other times challenging and inspirational. It has been central to rites of human sacrifice as well as the dedication of self-sacrificing behaviour of Saints.

With so much effort going into the search for answers to the questions of selfhood, we must ask first, what is the self? Here we find that there is no simple or easy answer, for again the consciousness seems to be at work to organize the many selves into the one and integrated working self.

We have such limited space and time that we cannot in detail look at all of the selves. We must limit ourselves to the body-image, the mind-image, the spiritual-image and the integrated composite: the self-image.

Our body-image gets started before birth and is well-developed before we are able to think or talk about it.[1] For that reason it has a powerful influence on our living because it is difficult to go back and examine some of the constituents of its development. A child lives entirely by its feelings in early stages of its existence. It is constantly dependent and therefore responsive to the feelings of those around it. Expressions of anger and disgust are so direct that the young child has no ready defence against them. Even utterances of disgust when changing a nappy may seep into a child's consciousness and impair feelings of self-worth. At that early stage the body becomes the focal point for most activity. Children that have been deprived of love, warmth and attention early in life tend to be hesitant and apprehensive, or over compensate these feelings by becoming aggressive and manipulative.[2] Often the feelings towards one's body become major factors in matters of illness and health.

Religious and cultural conditions also affect attitudes towards the body. For centuries those who denied feelings that were pleasurable and mortified the body were considered to be saints. In the puritan tradition denial of pleasure and good bodily feelings was as vigorous as the quest for good feelings among hedonists. Basically both positions are the same in their fear of bodily demands, fear of the effects of pleasure and fear of the failure to find pleasure. Basically the approach of modern medicine is puritanical in that it seeks to make the body behave according to laws that are set up as norms by those who practice biomedical disciplines. Jacob Needleman goes even further and says: 'It is . . . a mistake to think that modern medical science, including psychiatry, offers a relationship to the body significantly different from that of puritanism. The substitution of the love of pleasure for the hatred of pleasure means nothing here. It is all puritanism in a larger sense. The conflict between ego and nature remains'.[3]

If the body becomes a battleground for moral and behavioural problems the direct effect of conflict on body chemistry will impair immunological resources and prepare the way for uncontrolled viral growth and neoplastic tissue developments.[4] So instead of punishing the body or making it a centre of conflict, it seems important to value the body and treat it with care and consideration due 'the temple of God'. The best of the Christian tradition seeks to do that.

The mind image has developed with philosophical rationalism. René Descartes laid down the famous dictum, 'I think, therefore I am.' Instead of saying, 'I feel, therefore I am,' or 'I love, therefore I am,' or 'I believe, therefore I am,' he set the

43

stage for the ascendency of reason over emotion, human concern or faith. By discounting much of human experience by centring on the rational, he stimulated important advancement in science and philosophy at the cost of eliminating much human experience from a place in the scientific spectrum.

The research in psychosomatics has produced a major shift in emphasis. It has brought emotions back into the picture. If one hundred per cent of illness is psychosomatic in that it all involves both bodily manifestations and feelings about them, the danger is that the pendulum will swing too far in the other direction and the rational controls will be weakened. The common phrase, 'Oh, its all in your head' has been so prevalent that one physician in self-defence has written a book entitled *It is Not All in Your Head*. Here again the conflict of mini-systems calls out for a larger perspective on human experience.

While it is important to recognize that the mind-image is a major part of the perception of self, it can be distorted out of shape and become a hazard to the self that encourages it. To deny the self proper care because of an overdependence on the mini-system of reason could become but another verification of our need to live beyond any limited and limiting perspective. So it is that the limitations of Berkeleyan philosophy have baited the trap into which many Christian Scientists have fallen.

The spiritual image usually appears in one of two forms. There is the body that develops a spiritual dimension, or there is a spirit that manifests itself in physical form through a body. In the former the spirit appears to be less significant than the body and in the treatment of illness tends to put the body first and only if and when biomedical efforts fail resorts to the spiritual possibilities for healing. The latter tends to place emphasis on the spiritual nature of the potential of the human being and may seek healing through non-physical resources first and supplement them by other modes of intervention.

Recent decades have shown a shift away from such philosophies as mechanism and materialism and such psychologies as behaviourism and the conditioned response. This has opened the doors to a flood of systems and practices designed to free the spirit and develop the psychic nature of the individual. New cults and consciousness centring exercises are constantly being replaced by the newest fad. While some have a usefulness, many are but illustrations of the misleading character of mini-systems that claim much for little and usually lead to frustration and disillusionment.

Much of the energy of this spiritually focussed activity is directed towards health and healing. Often esoteric in nature and manipulative in method they seem more concerned about bringing people under the control of a mini-system that is helping them to discipline and direct the full resources of their inner being towards a wiser use of highly disciplined spiritual power. The mood of this genre is expressed in phrases like 'My guru is better than your guru.' Instead of stimulating genuine personal growth there is a tendency to foster immaturities and dependencies in combination with commitment that builds on trivial loyalties rather than on a systems view that can integrate spiritual energies as it provides adequate criteria for evaluating the mini-systems. Only then does it seem possible to bring together the best of modern research and experience in a pattern of discovery that will move towards the goals envisioned by Pierre Teilhard de Chardin, Simone Weil, Karl Menninger, Viktor Frankl and others who synthesize thought and feeling around spiritually challenging goals.

It seems that the time is propitious for a new maxi-system view of health that can capitalize on the spiritual interest now present and meld it with the research in psychosomatics and the willingness to explore new types of co-operation among the persons concerned with wise health care. The maxi-system we seek would achieve a self-image that brings together the most mature form of body-mind-spirit-image into a commitment to accept the challenges and commitments that go with the larger systems view emerging from new perceptions of wholeness of being in individual and society.

Resources useful in refining the skills and perceptions of the inner being have long been known and practised in various ways in different cultures. Usually those who practised the spiritual disciplines were a limited group sometimes set apart by society for the refinement of their special sensitivities. Every culture seems to have had its equivalent of monastic orders.

All seem to know that consciousness can be disciplined. When the practice of disciplined and sharply focussed thought is skilfully developed it extends the powers of the mind. Altered states of awareness appear to become the source of heightened psychic awareness so that in meditation integrative processes of thought can take place. So it is not unusual for people to see visions, experience mystical awareness and forms of spiritual sensitivity as they become skilful meditators. Researchers find that clairvoyance, clairsentience, clairaudience and telepathic communication are more common when the mind and spirit are engaged in spiritual discipline. Even out-of-body experiences occur as thresholds of consciousness are modified and these may be misinterpreted as levitation. Instead of these experiences being abnormal, they tend to show that the unused powers of consciousness when properly developed can extend the function of consciousness and enhance the spiritual activity of life.

The basic problem with much meditation is that it toys with the powers of consciousness without a theological or philosophical base adequate to set the boundaries within which these powers can be safely used. This tends towards the magical which violates the law and order of the universe rather than seeking disciplined co-operation with it. This again reflects the conflict of mini-systems rather than the revelation of a higher order that emerges as the fulfilment of an ordered approach to a maxi-system that brings together partial realities in a supreme reality. As Jesus put it, these quests for the magical and miraculous are efforts to tempt God. His effort was to reveal the higher spiritual order that put it all together rather than stimulating more conflict.

It is in this light that we are able to understand the concept of meditation and prayer that Jesus taught. It not only tells us something about the teaching of Jesus but it also tells us much about him. When the disciples sought to understand the power that was present in Jesus as he masterfully met life, they did not ask what was his philosophical system or psychological method. They did not ask where he found his apt illustrations of his deep wisdom. They seemed to know that all they observed was support by a back-up system that constantly empowered him. They traced this power to the discipline of life they observed when he rose early and went out to a quiet place to nurture the dimensions of his consciousness in an intimate relationship to the source of all power, the creative spirit of God. To this spirit he resonated. So they asked him what he did when he prayed so that they might learn the secret of his power.

The disciples of Jesus apparently never heard him engage in audible prayer because it was a very private thing. There is question among the scholars as to the authenticity of any of the recorded prayers found in the New Testament. Even the prayer usually referred to as the Lord's Prayer is apparently an insertion made during the time when the church was developing a liturgy and sought the warrant of Jesus to help establish this practice in the early church. Anyone reading that prayer as it is juxtaposed in the sixth chapter of Matthew will see that the verbal prayer contradicts the teaching admonitions that surround it. They emphasize the private rather than the corporate discipline of communication between creature and creator. They emphasize the fact that prayer never need ask of God, for God already knows the needs of the inner being. Jesus denied the uniqueness of the power he developed in prayer and affirmed that those who mastered the inner disciplines would do even greater things than he had been able to do. So he taught the development and nurture of the inner kingdom where the power of God could be discovered and developed. This was a use of the power of consciousness that was compatible with the nature of God and the nature of the universe as he understood and taught it. It brought together the revelation of God in the depths of the inner being as well as in the structure of the law and order at work in the universe.

How then are we to discover the nature of prayer as Jesus revealed it? We seek the basic principles he taught and personified. He made it quite evident to those who observed him that he put the disciplining of his spirit first in all things. It took precedence in his daily routine, in his way of thinking and in the things that he did. He paid attention to God first, foremost and constantly. This was the order of his life.

Another thing that Jesus taught about prayer both by precept and example was that this form of special communication was not something you did. Rather it was something you were through your whole being. This is quite a different concept of prayer from what we are usually taught and urged to employ. But how else can we interpret the admonition to pray without ceasing? It has to be a way of life rather than something added. Even Paul's idea of being constant in prayer implies this all-encompassing practice of an inner discipline that permeates all of life. It was a compelling purpose that dominated all the rest of living, a way of life. Perhaps we best understand the words about 'the way, the truth, and the life' when we think of them in terms of the spiritual discipline employed in this form of being in prayer and prayer in being.

Jesus also taught that prayer changes things. This idea at first seems to violate our strong commitment to the law and order of the universe, but then we remember the inventive-creative capacity within us that keeps our partnership with

48

God an ongoing concern. When we look at the idea more closely it becomes more comprehensible for if there is anything that our century has affirmed it is that thinking changes things. Scientists and engineers put their heads together and come up with earth-changing achievements. Within the lifetime of many now alive electric power, electronic communication, intercontinental flight, trips to the moon and probers of outer space along with laser surgery and powerful new drugs have become an accepted part of life, even commonplace. These things are evidence that thinking changes things. Prayer is a special type of thinking set free from material limits to stimulate and direct the most audacious assumptions of the inner being. Certainly it is quite reasonable to assume that this kind of specialized thinking will also have its impact on life. And the more valid the non-material realities become the more urgent becomes the need to understand and use prayer as a source of power to change things for the better, including the power to heal.

Prayer not only changes things. It changes people. When life is governed by an all-consuming urge to discover and implement the sources of spiritual power, it is inevitable that the seeker will be moulded into a different person with new values, new perspectives and new power to achieve spiritual goals. The lives of multitudes down through history attest the fact that a change in the focus of life produces fruits in abundance. The conversion experiences of Paul, St Francis, Ignatius Loyola, Martin Luther and John Wesley, just to mention a few, are examples of this power at work to change life. A new perspective made a new person.

Jesus also illustrated in his own life and in his teaching of others that this type of prayer is probably the most difficult thing a person will ever be called on to do. The discipline of his life led to a supreme form of self-sacrifice and he came to the place where in his praying he was so totally involved in an inner struggle that the scripture records that he sweat blood

49

(Luke 22.44). This type of prayer demands that the person move beyond all forms of self-deception and game-playing to confront the demands of the major systems view of life. This would be well beyond the escapes and excuses that are provided by the mini-systems we so easily create and to which we gladly give our limited and self-deceiving loyalty. Unwarranted anger can no longer pose as righteous indignation. Petty self-indulgence can no longer masquerade as human rights and justice. Self-deception can no longer claim to be psychic sensitivity. It requires that we come to terms with ourselves in the light of the highest and best we know, the revelation of God through the disciplines of the spirit made known to us in the teaching and life pattern of the example of loyalty to a systems approach to life that excluded no truth, and harboured no falsehood of body, mind or spirit.

How are these resources found in the teaching of Jesus about prayer made available to us? There is no one way. There may be many ways, in fact as many ways as there are people seeking the way, for there is always a personal dimension for nurturing the inner kingdom. Since I have retired I have been able to give time and effort to a high form of pastoral care that is implicit in the role of the spiritual guide or spiritual director. Here the method is to work closely with a person in quite individual terms, not to teach or manipulate but rather to share the growing edge of discovery about the inner being which is primarily concerned about the three non-material qualities of reality.

For fifteen years I have worked with these special seekers, mature men and women wanting more of life than they had so far found. Varied as a United Airline pilot, a medical director of an intensive care unit, a musician, clergymen of several denominations, scientists and researchers, nurses and teachers, they share a common interest in discovering a fuller aspect of their beings. With no effort to mould or compel their thinking and feelings I have tried to help them discover and nourish their unique genius for life. The adventure of this voyage of personal discovery has called for many hours of exploring the inner treasure of their beings waiting to be set free to grow to its fuller possibility.

It has been a rare privilege to watch the disciplined growth of the boundaries of being as new life patterns emerged, new value systems formed and new life-styles touched all of life with awe and wonder. Newly-discovered meanings were woven into a way of life, and worship became a cosmic relationship rather than an occasional act. The power within sought disciplined use of consciousness, the winsome invitation of meditation and the powerful perceptions of prayer created new meaning and purpose for life. The healing and redeeming love of the Holy Spirit became more than a phrase. Rather it became life itself. The self discovered its true nature. The power within burst through to new life. Like an atom brought to the place where it could release its great power, so the person realized the potential of self and made it actual. Yes, there are resources for disciplining the spirit. The partial images of the self become one image, and the power within became one power. Like the laser beam the intensified power of life was organized to work for one purpose, one system that encompasses all systems.

6

Mysticism

Learning how to discriminate, discipline and define the inner powers that are important to holistic healing is of the utmost importance. Let us look first at why mysticism is so difficult to bring into focus. The mystic usually feels the experience has such transcendent quality about it that something important would be lost if it were reduced to the limiting symbolism of words. In effect the mystic says, 'If you have had the experience no one could put it into words for you.' Usually the mystic would describe the experience as integrative. All of a sudden the conflicts of life are resolved, the mysteries dispelled and one realizes that all there is is one and indivisible. Usually the mystic would claim that the experience is esoteric, combining the profound, the secret and available only to those who are adequately prepared to confront and understand transcendent truth. This is why mystics often retreat into small groups or communities carefully selected by the keepers of the mysteries.

These special esoteric communities have been non-Christian as well as Christian. From the very beginning of the Christian era they have presented a problem because their loyalty to the non-material made them potential allies while their value system often turned them into subtle enemies. In their use of psychic resources they often confused undisciplined people who tried to combine psychic power with limited theological and psychological perspectives. St Paul had some trouble with those who confused the mystery religions with Christian teaching. In fact the Eastern Orthodox churches are still strongly influenced by a deep-rooted mysticism that sets them apart from the more materialistically-oriented churches in the Western tradition.

When I was living in Greece for several months and doing some lecturing at the Eastern Orthodox Seminary in Corinth, I decided to spend a night in the ruins of the Temple at Eleusis, a centre of the mystery religions. After studying the rites and rituals related to the worship of Demeter, I choose a clear, moonlit night and drove along the Via Sacra to the Temple. It was quiet and I was quite alone in a place that was some distance from any human habitation. Choosing a stately column at the end of the ruins where I could see the whole platform of the worship area I settled down for an evening's contemplation. I had been told that the very atmosphere was charged with spiritual energy. After hours of meditation I was unable to claim any special happening but there was a wonderful sense of peace as I tried to recreate in my imagination the rituals of death and resurrection that were central to their faith. While nothing unique to the place occurred it was far from a wasted evening and night for my consciousness was stimulated to noble thoughts and valued feelings.

Rare dimensions of consciousness have long existed. The wonder of consciousness has been a privilege that separates the human from other forms of life, but it has also been an almost intolerable burden for it places heavy demands upon life without making clear the boundaries within which that special endowment can be wisely employed. Perhaps we best understand the Christian revelation as the maxi-system that makes it possible for us to employ the privileges of consciousness without being misled for the boundaries that are often uncertain and confusing are made firm in their discipline that Christian goals make clear. Yet like other traditions, the burden and the privilege have often been confused and the historical and contemporary practices within Christendom verify the difficulty in using the power within the boundaries that would best define its usefulness.

Let us look briefly at some of the manifestations of the mixing of mystical power with mini-systems that carry within the seeds of their own inadequacy and self-destruction. There is anti-intellectual mysticism, anti-materialistic mysticism and scientific mysticism. Each verifies a part of the truth emerging from individual and collective human experience but each seems to have limited its usefulness by binding its perceptions to an inadequate theological and philosophical system. This not only impairs its fullest usefulness but has often become a devisive and reductionist force compromising its ultimate goal by its loyalty to the claims of a mini-system.

Let us look first at anti-intellectual mysticism. One of the major trends in non-material interest in recent years has been the anti-intellectual mood of Eastern philosophies. Following Herman Hesse's *Journey to The East*,[1] many persons have shown an active interest in this contemporary form of trans-cendentalism. Zen is a popular expression of this mood. With its confounding expression it has invited people to turn away from intellectualisms to find meaning in the apparently meaningless.

The preoccupation with the purely rational which involves the rejection of people and feelings has brought the world to the brink of extinction. The power of science to create destructive power without adequate restraints in politics and social patterns has shaken faith in both science and the intellect. The inverse of faith in science and the intellect is to move towards the non-intellectual. The problem is that like a rudderless ship the power of consciousness uncontrolled can produce inanities. 'The secret of Zen is Zen's secret.' Profound or inane? 'When you sit in meditation it is not the thinking about God or the dwelling on divine reality or the striving for your better self that should possess you. It is simply the sitting . . . When I raise my hand thus, that is Zen. But when I assert that I have raised my hand, Zen is no more there.' This effort to assert the primary of being itself passes a judgment on cause-effect processes. 'The Christian seems always to be doing something because . . . Because he should do a good deed, he does . . . He is a response to a "because factor". He may not believe in all these "becauses", but he feels a sense of guilt if he does not act as if he believed them. Hence, he can never truly be himself.'[2] It is impossible to try to catch the nature of Zen in a few words, but at least we get some flavour of its anti-intellectual mood. It may well be a valid judgment in our inadequate value system, but in itself it has the limitations of any mini-system that excludes one reality to emphasize another.

Within the main line tradition of Christendom there has been just as vigorous a form of anti-intellectualism. Often the emphasis of Pentecostals has been to avoid anything that they think stands in the way of the free action of the spirit. So they advise their young people not to seek higher education because the nurturing of the intellect will automatically impair the nurture of the spirit. Avoid the critical study of the scriptures because that will prevent the Holy Spirit from speaking directly from its pages, for one form of truth is assumed to be in conflict with another. Similarly to employ a practitioner of biomedical healing is a sign of lack of faith and will prevent the kind of healing that comes from the unquestioned devotion to the power of intercessory prayer. I have worked with charismatics enough to know that their sincere devotion to a compelling mini-system often drives them to extremes of devisiveness and conflict. Often this produces an escape from the larger reality they need to face. To say, 'Since I have the baptism of the spirit I am free and I go my way and the rest of the family go theirs. I don't need them anymore because Jesus means everything to me,' may give escape from troublesome family relations but it provides a poor basis for confronting and resolving those problems. So the problems are not solved. A mini-system takes over and the anti-intellectual focus ill serves the needs for personal growth.

A significant segment of the Christian community in the West now professes loyalty to this type of mini-system. The misfortune is that the energy and discipline directed towards the mini-system stands as a barrier to the discipline and understanding that could make available the greater benefits of the systems view that marshals the resources of consciousness to bring the fruits of all realities into accessibility to the human mind, body and spirit. My stay in Japan where Zen is prevalent made me aware of both the winsomeness and the hazard of any mini-system, oriental or western, that compromises consciousness and its privileged but burdensome function.

Anti-materialistic mysticism shares some of the methods and practices of the anti-intellectual. More specifically rooted in Indian philosophies of the achievement of the good life by the denial of desires, these ideas in contemporary form appeal to those who have a compulsion to renounce the world and its temptations. Things become unimportant as emotional energies are turned inwards. Instead of striving for possessions that fail to provide satisfaction and breed only frustration, these ideas appeal to the young who have had a glut of things but a paucity of love and meaning for life. With shaved heads and simple attire, plus a master who has an answer for every question in return for absolute loyalty, these youth turn their backs on a way of life that has provided little satisfaction. In its place they make a commitment with absolute devotion to themselves and a cause that at last gives meaning to selfhood. So again a mini-system shows its power over life.

The visible assault on the values of capitalism is not unrecognized as these children of capitalist economics, education and value systems make their living witness against it. So capitalism as one mini-system fights against those who witness against it. With an ingenuity that was peculiar to the melding of the transcendentalism of Emerson and the capitalist interests of society, Mary Baker Eddy provided an interesting alternative for anti-materialistic mysticism. Using the philosophy of Bishop Berkeley which emphasized the reality of the sensory instead of the material she developed a system of thought and healing that denied the reality of illness and disease and claimed it was an error of mortal mind. In her book[3] *Science and Health* she developed a philosophical base, a form of self-discipline, and an organizational structure. She provided a form of denial that was peculiarly suited to the values of capitalism. Though she found it easier to preach than to practice, she built for herself a fortune and for her followers a focus for their loyalty. Supported now by energy physics and research in psychosomatics it would be assumed that Christian Science would have special appeal, but such does not seem to be the case. A major falling away appears to be taking place perhaps due to a more general understanding of cause-effect processes plus the prevalence of other forms of eastern mysticism.

The Christian Science approach to healing seems to be quite the opposite of the teaching of Jesus. He never denied illness, its presence or its reality. Rather he affirmed the power of faith as a larger reality so significant that it could produce a positive effect to modify bodily conditions. Here again we see the difference between a mini-system approach to reality in contrast to a larger view that integrates life at the same time that it makes room for all reality to function within a person free from conflict.

The mini-system of Christian Science seems to have found a way into some of the mainstream churches through the effort to create an either/or dichotomy rather than a both/and integration. Meeting with prayer groups around the country I find the idea expressed quite often that if people want to be healed through some form of spiritual agency they must eschew any and all other forms of healing. In effect they say, 'If you go to the physician you show you really don't believe in prayer so don't ask us to pray for you, O ye of little faith.' Instead of assuming that the power of God to heal may be manifest in many ways, the exclusiveness of the mini-system tends to assert that its way and its way only can claim validity. As is usually the case the mini-systems have a built-in premise that is God-limiting.

As we look at anti-intellectual and anti-materialistic mysticism we see that they have incorporated some demonstrable truths but have excluded a larger truth. Unfortunately there is an assumption that is unwarranted, for as all truth is one there need be no areas of conflict, only areas of misinterpretation.

Scientific mysticism has played an important role in the history of Christianity. While the organized church with its materialistic interest has not always been comfortable with the phenomena of science, it has provided an essential base for the work of scientists by believing in the basic dependability of the cosmic order, and the validity of the mind's ability to perceive truth. Without such ideas science would be set adrift.

Yet again and again in history when science moved too rapidly or challenged some facet of the mini-system of the church there was open conflict. So Giordano Bruno, a priest, was burned at the stake for preaching the heliocentric concept of the solar system. Galileo was obliged to recant his teaching about the universe gained from his telescopic probes of space because they were unacceptable to the church. The truths of Darwin and Freud were not accepted with open arms by churchmen. Even in our day the writings of Pierre Teilhard de Chardin were kept under wraps until after his death.

What has been true of the church has also been true of science. Partisanship among scientists has not been unknown. When Ignace Semmelweiss propounded his view of childbirth fever, other members of the medical profession ridiculed the possibility that disease could be transmitted by unseen organisms on the doctor's hands, which should be carefully scrubbed before touching a patient. Poor Dr Semmelweiss was actually hounded out of his mind and his profession and died destitute in an insane asylum. More recently, physicists ridiculed the claim of Pierre and Marie Curie that there were radioactive elements that could be isolated and used medically. After they had suffered much harrassment and rejection, their discoveries have become basic to modern physics and useful in therapeutic intervention. In 1916 Albert Abrams, a West Coast physician, wrote a book[4] showing how electronic devices could be used in medical diagnosis and treatment. He was accused of being a quack, lost his licence in California and was obliged to leave the country to practice in Canada. Now electrocardiagrams and electroencephalograms are constantly used in diagnosis and electromedical equipment is the basis for a highly sophisticated branch of medical intervention. The Committee for the Scientific Investigations of Claims of the Paranormal tried to give status to prejudice by rejecting the claims philosophically before investigating them scientifically.

An important insight that has emerged in recent years is that a technique, in and of itself, is inadequate to become the basis for a philosophy. Freud was always restless with his materialistic philosophy because it did not support his clinical findings, but he was a creature of his time and bound by its prevailing perspectives.[5] So biomedical practice has often been limited by its effort to extrapolate a philosophy from an accumulation of laboratory reports or a mass of clinical observation. Neo-Freudians have been searching for years for a more adequate base for interpreting the phenomena of human motivation and the power within that is constantly being observed in the most stringent of clinical settings.

Yet for centuries it has been clear within science that the scientist not only can be a mystic but inevitably must be. A scientist becomes a metaphysician as soon as he contemplates meaning and purpose. Blaise Pascal was a sound scientist and a Christian mystic. Emanuel Swedenborg was a scientist, philosopher, theologian and mystic. In his classic book *The Metaphysical Foundations of Modern Physical Science*,[6] Edwin Burtt shows the relationship of spiritual assumptions to the emergence of contemporary physical theory. Albert Einstein wrote a little book he called *Cosmic Religion*.[7] At the end of his *Scientific Autobiography* Max Planck cries, 'On to God'.[8]

In fact, both humanist psychology and energy physics may best be described as mystical systems. They use esoteric language that can be understood only by those initiated into the system. They deal with phenomena that can never be reduced to material or sensory data but must use the symbolic language of mathematical formulae. They work towards a unified field theory which assumes that all there is is one and that ultimately all energy forms including the energy of consciousness will achieve compatible relationships. Towards this end physicists and psychologists now are working out the next steps in perception that will make the maxi-system comparable with various scientific concepts of reality at the same time that they are compatible with the ultimate form of human response in the activity of mystical awareness as the highest level of consciousness, what psychologists refer to as super-conscious manifestation.

During recent years I have been working with Henry Margenau, Sterling Professor of Physics at Yale, to try to isolate the unique energy of consciousness. His massive tome, *The Nature of Physical Reality* is a classic. In a recent letter he wrote, 'Much reading in modern biology has led me to conclude that ordinary Darwinism with its reliance on chance is insufficient to account for the facts of evolution, that elements of purpose, goal-directedness and even beauty enter the scene. It now appears to me that a postulate of the action of some Universal Consciousness will become inevitable and is compatible with modern science . . . I believe that in a universal sense that is above time, all events are present and real now. If you please, all future and past existence is uniquely on record, firmly engraved in timeless essence, or as some would say, in the mind of Universal Consciousness.'[9] So in these words of a leading philosopher of science we already see the acceptance of a contemporary scientifically approved maxi-system that moves beyond space and time and into the mind of the Universal Consciousness.

So we have three types of mysticism seeking a maxi-system essential to their completeness. The small approaches of anti-intellectual mysticism, or anti-materialistic mysticism or even mini-scientific perspectives are not adequate for where we are today in science and the healing arts. Consciousness cannot realize or express its full power in a world of restraints imposed by mini-systems. It needs a cosmic dimension where the highest level of human consciousness resonates with what Dr Margenau calls the Universal Consciousness. Now is the time to break free and realize what Pierre Teilhard de Chardin envisioned, a spiritual being moving towards an Omega point where all forms of truth are integrated in the Noosphere, a realm where the spiritual realities dominate life and bring it to its fulfilment.[10]

Learning from Historical Perspectives

Interest in health care has deep roots in the past. Archaeologists find evidence of rather skilled surgery in the trepanied skulls of ancient peoples. That some of the surgery was successful is shown by the evidences of healing that survived with the skulls.

Anthropologists in their study of primitive societies almost always record the special role of the healer who seemed to combine magic, herbal knowledge and psychological wisdom as resources in serving the health needs of the people in his culture.

Medical historians explore the practices of ancient India and China and find well-developed modes of health care and forms of preventive medicine that may be equal to or superior to practices in our day.

Early forms of medical practice always seem to be closely related to the philosophy or theology that was prevalent in the culture. People interpreted health and illness in ways that were compatible with their sense of selfhood and their perception of the cosmic processes around them. As illness and injury were experienced they usually gave it meaning in one or another of three ways.

First was the response of animism where everything was alive with spiritual energy. If you offended a rock its spirit might respond in such a way that it would fall and cause you injury. If you offended the spirit of a snake or an animal it might bite you. If you climbed a tree and the limb broke it could have been because the spirit of the tree was violated by the invasion of its sacred precincts. The basic philosophy provided the cause-effect understanding that gave meaning to the experience. The form of intervention might be to make a sacrifice designed to calm the angered feelings of the offended spirit lurking in every object of nature.

The second way was to attribute a religious meaning to the events of life. If God was all powerful, then all that happened was attributable to divine agency. God was the one and only cause. When something good happened it was obvious that God was pleased. If something tragic or painful happened it was obvious that God was offended and the offender was being punished for the misdeed. Punishment and illness were closely related in such a system. There was even question as to whether it was propitious to interfere with God's punishment by trying to ameliorate the pain and suffering of the diseased and injured. In some traditions it was more specifically an act of interference with the karmic intent of divine process.

Third was magic, mystery and the miraculous. The known was surrounded by a world of the unknown and unknowable. The mysterious realm could be penetrated only by one who was entrusted with the keys to the mysteries. Those who possessed a psychic endowment seemed to have a key to the mysteries. Through magical incantations and esoteric practices the medicine men were able to exert control over the forces that affected good and evil, illness and health. Perhaps the early roots of rites, rituals and ceremonies are found in human efforts to control the forces of the natural and supernatural that are manifest in human suffering. Special people did special things to try to achieve special effects. So a priesthood was born.

Yet even early in the efforts to discover the meaning of illness and disease there were indications that there was some understanding of the cause-effect processes operative. If certain things were done it was possible to ward off the offending forces of nature. So amulets were worn to ward off illness. Understanding of elemental aspects of nutrition show-ed up in warnings to avoid foods that were poisonous while the eating of strength-giving foods was encouraged.

Perhaps the best known ancient health code is found in the laws of Moses or the Deuteronomic code. In the book of the Levis, the priests are entrusted with the religious, civil and health laws of the Jewish people. Apparently made up of primitive taboos chapters eleven to fifteen reflect practices that seem unnecessarily harsh and cruel. While in terms of modern medical insight they offer little that is useful, in their own primitive way they indicate that much time and attention as well as applied insight was attached to health care. Not only do they explore physical symptoms of bodily disturbance, but also they are alert to the unfortunate impact on life of perverted forms of behaviour and maladaptive emotional responses.

The Levitican law warns against behaviour that could spread disease. This early code orders careful cleansing of anything touched by the diseased person, even to the destroying of the dishes from which he has eaten. Instead of signs saying 'Spitting Prohibited' the code says, 'If he who has the discharge spits on one who is clean, then he shall wash his clothes and bathe himself in water.'

The code provides harsh measures of quarantine. 'The priest shall shut up the person with the itching disease for seven days' (Lev. 13.33). 'The Lord said to Moses, "Command the people of Israel that they put out of the camp every leper and every one having a discharge"' (Num. 5.1). The leper is separated from the community and marked as a social hazard: 'He shall wear torn clothes and let the hair of his head hang loose, and he shall cover his upper lip and cry "unclean, unclean" . . . and he shall dwell alone in a habitation outside the camp' (Lev. 13.45).

In addition to numerous preventive measures charged to them, the priests have an important role in what might be considered therapeutic intervention. This would include ritual sacrifice. Magical numbers were used when a diseased person would be sprinkled with blood seven times and then bathed in the Jordan seven times. The idea of the scapegoat that developed then still has relevance in a scapegoat theology that blames tragedy and illness on God and then curses God as recommended by Job's wife (Job 2.9). The code orders that the priest 'shall lay both his hands upon the head of a live goat and confess over him all the iniquities of the people . . . and he shall put them upon the head of the goat, and send them away into the wilderness . . . The goat shall bear all their iniquities upon him into a solitary land' (Lev. 16.21). The psalmist probably refers to this practice of ritualized forgiveness when he says, 'As far as the east is from the west, so far does he remove our transgressions from us' (Ps. 103).

As is apt to be the case in times of change and transition, apparently contradictory ideas are put side by side. In this Jewish code there are remnants of the appeal to magic and the rituals that are employed to produce magical results. Combined with them are the evidences of recognition of the laws of cause and effect and the concern to operate in relation to them. This was especially useful of preventive measures taken to ward off diseases that were assumed to be contagious.

It was in this context of more rational approaches to disease that works of mercy and acts of compassion began to be observed. While it was still believed that pain and suffering could be warning signs given by God to make people aware of the meaning of their behaviour, it was also within the bounds of reason to bind up wounds, pour on oil and water and care for the injured. At this point it became increasingly clear that the person who was injured and helpless became at least temporarily a ward of the family or the community.

Implicit in the ancient Jewish practices is an awareness of the fact that attitudes are related to health. Social codes place restraints on individuals. When the individual breaks the social limitations there is apt to be guilt. The guilt may cause anxiety and apprehension and these affect organic function.

Thus guilt and forgiveness are related to illness and health. So also the image of personal integrity is related to health. 'Blessed is the man who sweareth to his own hurt and changeth not' (Ps. 15.4). 'What doth the Lord require of thee but to do justly, love mercy and walk humbly with your Lord?' (Micah 6.8). 'A lying tongue and hands that shed innocent blood are an abomination' (Deut. 21.9). Ancient writ defines actions which violate the order of integrity and justice as unacceptable to God and community. Unless the individual is able to purge his being of such acts of aggression, perfidy and disloyalty his social status is insecure and his health is in jeopardy. Holistic approaches are built in as the social structure recognizes the cause-effect processes at work in individual and community life.

In the New Testament we have a great leap forward. No longer is God thought of as a capricious being easily manipulated by burnt offerings and animal sacrifices. In the place of magical concepts and manipulative rituals there is a dependable universe of cause-effect laws as the revelation of God and the obligation to live with personal responsibility to the power of God that is available to those who discipline their inner being to be responsive to it. In this quantum leap ahead in theological thinking Jesus stands as a watershed between the thought of the past and the thought of the future.

The popular view of Jesus as a healer indicates the need for healing and the concerns about health in his day. Yet it is equally clear that Jesus did not want a preoccupation with physical healing to obscure his purpose. He proclaimed a way of life that involved far more than physical healing alone. He sought to enunciate a quality of right relationship with God that would permeate all of life, body, mind and spirit. So again and again when people were healed he sought to avoid publicity and urged them to tell no man (Matt. 8.4; Mark 8.26, 30; 9.9; Luke 5.14).

The Gospel record refers to some seventy incidents of

66

personal or group healing with varying degrees of elaboration. The accounts are quite limited but even the brief ones indicate various methods were employed. Sometimes the patient was not physically present and intercessory prayer seems to have been the major resource. And at other times there was laying on of hands and tactile forms of communication as they touched Jesus or he touched them. At other times this was supplemented by counselling with a major modification of attitude on the part of the sick person. At other times Jesus appears to make a salve of the chemically rich soil of the region and apply it directly to the afflicted part.

From the limited records we have it appears that Jesus used several different philosophical assumptions in his approach to healing. He recognized the impact of heredity where affliction could be passed on from generation to generation. He recognized the influence of circumstance when innocents suffered from conditions over which they had no control. He recognized the impact of evil forces in the world, both political and social. He recognized the personal processes that involved cause and effect where people created the situations from which they suffered. He also recognized the common symptoms of communicable diseases such as fevers and leprosy.

Jesus never denied the existence of illness or disease. He did not treat it as illusion. He did not practice denial. Rather he recognized and used spiritual, psychological and religious resources that usually overcame symptoms and disturbed states of being. However, he worked within a social milieu that had its impact even upon him and his works. The scripture reports that in Nazareth where doubt, suspicion and reductionist practices were prevalent he did no mighty works (Mark 6.5).

Jesus did not refer to what he did as miraculous. He seemed to prefer the term 'mighty works' (Matt. 11.20, 13.58). In his ministry he was firmly committed to the law and order processes at work in the universe, where for every cause there was an effect and for every effect a cause. He perceived God not as capricious but as utterly dependable. His temptations in the desert centred around his discovery of the disciplines that could work within that law and order structure. He was committed to obeying God's laws and would abridge none of them. He would not violate molecular structure to make stone into bread for man does not live by bread alone. He would not break the laws of gravity and inertia by jumping from the mantle of the temple to make a spectacular soft landing because he would not tempt God to violate his own law. Nor would he engage in political compromise where he sacrificed half of humanity in order to gain easy ascendency over the other half because he was committed to serving God only (Luke 4). The law and order of God's creation was sacred to Jesus and he disciplined himself to work within those laws.

A theology of responsibility to God's law is basic to health care because it seeks to discover and work with the laws of physical, mental and spiritual wholeness and holism. The cosmological base from which Jesus operated made no room for playing fast and loose with the revelation of God. Rather it was his purpose to achieve the strenuous discipline that could wisely work within the framework of God's creation. He refused to work within the limits of a small sized tribal idea of God. There are no limits on God and no analogies are fitting for God is not like anything. God is. Jesus echoes some of the concepts of Job who saw God in his infinite majesty and power, his creative wisdom and eternal providence (Job 38, 39, 40).

How did Jesus and the New Testament perceive God? Usually the reference is to forms of energy that can be translated into continued revelation by the works of the Holy Spirit. God is light and in him is no darkness at all. Light is the raw material of all creation, the first form of energy from which all else emerges (I John 1.5). God is power, the manifestation of that creation in natural form, the ultimate purpose of Jesus to reveal the power to become children of God and joint heirs with him (John 1.12). Truth is the intellectual or scientific dimension of God's creative nature that Jesus revealed. I am the way, the truth and the life (John 14.17; 17.17). God is Spirit, the non-material processes that resonate to God's nature. God is spirit and those who worship him must worship him in spirit and in truth (John 4.24). God is love and they that dwell in love abide in him. This is the emotional commitment that responds positively to all of the other forms of God's power and presence. This is the activating force in human life (Matt. 5.45).

Jesus refused to limit God by human forms of judgment. We cannot play games with God and his laws. We cannot break God's laws though we may break ourselves against them. God does not play favourites, for his judgment is beyond human judgments. His sun shines on the good and evil and his rain falls on the just and unjust (John 4.8). The God he revealed and worshipped was not man-made or man-manipulated but rather was discovered by searching humans, revealed by disciplined humanity and fulfills our deepest needs as we pay attention to God more devotedly than to anything on earth. His revelation of God is the highest that has ever been perceived. It demands so much in human commitment that we often try to reduce the revelation. Yet the form of responsibility and discipline implicit in accepting the revelation is essential to meeting the highest demands of a healing ministry such as his.

In his teaching and in his self-disciplined revelation Jesus provided a philosophical base for holistic health. It is relevant to our day. Ours may be the first generation in history that has a psychological base and a cosmological concept compatible with the revelation of the New Testament. We may be the ones who are able to understand what the New Testament was trying to make known to humankind. Our concerns about health and healing may open the doors to a more valid theological perception for our day and the days that are ahead.

Certainly the disciples were inadequately prepared to develop the concepts of God and creation that Jesus revealed. There is every evidence from the scriptures that Good Friday and Easter were hardly past before the disciples were engaged in the task of reducing the ideas of Jesus to fit the psychology and cosmology of their day. They had lived all their lives with the Ptolmaic idea of 'out there' and 'up there'. So they tried to materialize the person of Jesus in this limited view of creation with ascension upward towards a geographical plateau above the earth. Similarly they tried to reduce the nature of the human to the symbolic forms that were not unrelated to the prevalent Aristotelian idea of the human as refined animal form. This idea shows up at Pentecost where the Holy Spirit descends from above to touch human flesh and activate it from above with a descending dove or tongues of fire. With this thinking the human being was first a body and then a spirit, rather than first being made in the image of God and then given a bodily form subsequently and temporarily (Acts 2).

We can have deep sympathy for the disciples for they have not been alone in their reductionist activities. The church through the centuries has been far more comfortable with a materialistic starting point for approaching the revelation of Jesus than it has been in developing spiritual resonance to a spiritual revelation. Yet there is little warrant for us to limit our movement into the future by their inadequacies when they no longer need to be ours. A theological stance that recognizes the full spiritual potential of each human may be far more useful in a holistic maxi-system than a limited and limiting form of reductionism.

The early church gave an important place to healing. Apparently one of the major roles of the elders of the church was to engage in individual and ritualized forms of healing. Yet here the emphasis seemed to be more on magic and miraculous rather than a realization of disciplined spiritual living. Indirectly they implied some understanding of the use of spiritual power, for they seemed to realize that the prayers of the righteous or spiritually disciplined had greater efficacy (James 5.17).

The disciples and the members of the early church were able to do significant works of healing under the power of the Holy Spirit (Acts 4.29–31). However, they seemed to attribute their achievements to miraculous intervention from above rather than the disciplined response from the inner kingdom of power they were admonished by Jesus to nurture (Luke 17.21). So the nurture of the inner kingdom was ignored or neglected and the power centre grew in the material structure of the church.

For centuries Christendom was organized about a strong institution that was invested with special power through the administering of sacraments. The seven basic sacraments exerted magical power from birth to death by saving babies from hell, changing bread to flesh, and making sure of safe entry into the realm of divine grace at death. Transubstantiation and supersubstantiation exerted powerful influence over the lives of people as it enhanced the role of the institution in life. The transfer of emphasis from the inner to the outer kingdom was soon completed and for centuries this continued. The Reformation worked to bring major changes. When the significance of the inner kingdom was reduced the significance of the human being suffered with it. This laid the basis for biomedical authority rather than the holistic approach to health. The possibility for continued revelation through individuals was reduced and the power of the institution flourished as its power over spiritual matters was consolidated. Political, social and economic matters became more important than the nourishing of the spirit that dwelt within. When the church used people rather than nourishing their inner beings all humankind suffered.

Institutional power was preserved through monastic orders that compelled absolute subservience to the order. This tended to limit the possibility for continued revelation of spiritual insight by individuals. Significant breakthrough did emerge here and there with individuals; St Francis, St Theresa and St John of the Cross. Yet here it seemed to be dependent upon the unusual psychic gifts of the individual that broke through institutional restraints. These were usually opposed by the church that feared mysticism. The Franciscan order was penetrated by agents of the Vatican and its character changed. A whole crusade was needed to mercilessly destroy the Cathori with their unrestrained commitment to spirituality rather than institutional authority.

However, in structured form the works of health care were performed by such orders as the Sisters of Mercy, the followers of St Bernard and the hospices set up to care for pilgrims, crusaders and other travellers. Some of the practices now being preserved by the Hospice movement are rooted in the ideas developed by medical orders that ministered to the sick and wounded by works of compassion and loving care.

With the emergence of research in medicine, the study of anatomy and the more objective study of the phenomena of illness and health, the church became a sponsor of hospitals. This role was shared as we now have three types of treatment centres. Most cities have church-related hospitals which still exert a philosophical influence on medical practice. For instance, one would not likely go to a Catholic hospital for an abortion. A second type of hospital is sponsored, financed and controlled by the municipality within which it functions: the city hospital. Another type of socially-administered hospital is state or federally maintained and supported. These are usually hospitals for the mentally ill, veteran's administration facilities or military treatment centres. In each there tend to be mixtures of philosophical assumptions that emerge from religious, scientific or materialistic assumptions. The long influence of the church is being modified in contemporary health care practices.

It is interesting to note that with the growing influence of holistic perceptions the base for philosophical exploration has come full circle. The material that is activated by the spirit is increasingly becoming the spirit that is exerting its influence over the material. In our next chapter we will explore this trend more fully. Here let us recapitulate what we have noted in the brief historical survey of this chapter.

In the long, slow evolution of health care practices there has usually been a strong non-material or spiritual influence. Even in the most primitive approaches to health care in animism, the works of early medicine men, and in ancient health codes, illness and disease were never considered to be merely physical or organic. Other essentially non-physical or spiritual forces were assumed to be at work. It has been only in recent centuries that there was conflict between the material and spiritual. In the Middle Ages it was not incompatible to believe that there were two sources of legitimate evidence, revelation and reason. Revelation guided people in understanding the spiritual realm just as reason guided people in exploring the objective, measurable world of material things. With Descartes' contribution to philosophy the methods of reason flourished and science made great strides ahead. Reason was so effective in shaping progress that revelation was outmoded and suspect. The materialistic premise was fixed in the dictum that whatever exists exists in some quantity and therefore can be measured. Soon the corollary emerged that if it cannot be measured it is a reasonable assumption that it does not exist.[1]

The impact of this assumption on medical practice is clear. 'In its pursuit of objectivity, medical science has grown relatively insensitive to the less measurable qualities of human life. Quantitative laboratory information generally takes precedence over assessment of a patient's emotional life or even over balanced clinical judgment.'[2] Thus contemporary med-

73

ical researchers pass judgment on their own attitudes, practices and philosophical assumptions.

Now from within the laboratory the persistent research into the sources of illness keeps running into the non-objective aspects of human life. Illness is seen more and more as a language of the body trying to say something that has its own unique importance to those who will listen carefully. These subjective forces keep asserting themselves powerfully and are busily at work to question the adequacy of purely objective approaches to human illness and disease. In fact from within medical research itself come the strongest evidences of the need to restore the subjective to its proper place in the understanding of the cause-effect processes at work in illness and health.

This being the case, let us then turn our explorations towards the laboratory material and medical research that appears to be in active conflict with the more prevalent assumptions of biomedical practice.

8

A Broadening Awareness

One of the most logically compelling, and from the point-of-view of the medical establishment, most threatening developments in contemporary medicine has been the rapid growth of psychosomatic research. The basic assumption of this form of research is that the person develops the malady so the study of the patient in all the aspects of life is important to elicit the sources of the disturbance. While this perspective is not new, it is almost inevitable that its implications have been resisted because they are based on assumptions quite different from those of traditional medicine.

An article in a recent issue of a medical journal[1] delineated the main assumptions of biomedical philosophy as follows:

- Disease is avoidable
- Disease is undesirable
- Every disease is caused by a lesion
- The only admissible evidence is objective evidence
- Health professionals are the best providers of health needs
- Medical problems have medical solutions
- Increased demands for health care can be met by greater numbers of health professionals
- The more health care received, the greater the chance of health
- Health care is a right

Psychomatic research and its findings challenge each of these assumptions. When and how did the interest in psychosomatics and psychogenics start? It has been around a long time as an unorganized awareness. First it emerged from large amounts of generalized perception on the part of medical practitioners. Physicians puzzled by a patient's ailment and uncertain as to the specific medicine to be prescribed often used an unspecific and inert substance to see what would happen. They found that the patient often responded positively to the inert substance or sugar pill. Something else was at work in the patient. Interest in this something else gave rise to research in the placebo response.

Similarly, physicians found that bedside manner had an effect. Tender loving care and just being there had an effect. Called in the middle of the night, a physician would find on reaching the bedside that the patient was relaxed, in less pain and also apologetic for calling. Reduction of anxiety and the promise of medical attention had produced positive results. All of these things had been known for a long time but the meaning had not been objectively explored.

Dr Walter Cannon, a professor at Harvard Medical School, looked into this unexplored patient response. He came up with some interesting findings. He had long been interested in the role of the glandular system as that part of the body that most immediately responded to emotional stress. He developed the concept of homeostasis as the chemically stable condition of the body. Temporary emotional stress produced immediate but short term modification of body chemistry as it stimulates the glands, the body's chemical factories. Chronic emotional stress produced long term chemical change. This was manifest by a generalized breakdown of the immune resources of the body, for when there was loss of the body defences the homeostatic balance within the body was impaired and disease or abnormal cell division could run rampant. Dr Cannon wrote two books that had great influence. In the first he reported research on bodily responses to various forms of emotional excitation.[2] In the second he explored the glandular system and how it works homeostatically.[3] With objective research these pioneering books clearly established the relationship of strong feelings and bodily responses. Medical science has never been quite the same since. While it could resist such insights, it could not completely ignore them.

Shortly after the Cannon studies, a remarkable physician who was unusually well-qualified for the task through her work in psychology, medicine, psychiatry and religion, set about bringing together for the first time a comprehensive study of the relation of emotions to the etiology of illness and disease. Published in 1935[4] and revised several times her work has become the classic study on the subject. Flanders Dunbar's book has 263 pages of notes and more than 5000 bibliographical references. It has been the cornerstone for additional research as well as modified assumptions in exploring the sources of illness and disease.

Dr Dunbar also thought of illness in new ways. Instead of disease being a breakdown of a mechanical piece of equipment it was seen as a unique language form, the body trying to tell anyone who would listen something significant about what was happening to it. The role of the physician was changed as different questions were asked. Instead of 'What can we do to modify these symptoms?', the more important question became, 'What is this body condition trying to tell us?' As dreams are the metaphor of the unconscious, so illness and disease become the metaphors of the body. In her book Dr Dunbar examines carefully a variety of human ailments and attempts to decipher the metaphoric language that is implicit in the body's specialized utterance.

Dr Dunbar seeks to translate the body language of each organ system. Starting with the nervous system, she moves to the musculature, the glandular system, general metabolism and heat regulation, cardiovascular system, respiratory organs and gastrointestinal systems, genito-urinary and gastrointestinal systems, sensory organs, the skin and the skeleton.

77

She even mentions the diseases physicians create through the power of their suggestions and the patients who make doctors ill by their stubborn resistance to every effort to stimulate the healing process. In each body system she finds evidence of the sometimes desperate effort of the body to communicate its needs and conditions. She feels that the physician should become an expert in listening to and understanding the eloquent language of the body.

As a result of the work of Dr Dunbar, the concept of intropsychic balance was developed and the specialization of psychosomatic medicine had come of age. Yet even in the medical community the definitions that are essential are misused and misinterpreted. For instance, in a comprehensive medical encyclopaedia[5] the word psychogenic nowhere appears and the word psychosomatic is incorrectly used. People who work in holistic health need to use terms like placebo response, homeostasis, intropsychic balance, psychosomatic and psychogenic with accuracy and clear comprehension.[6] Building on the work of Cannon and Dunbar a group of researchers have added significantly to our understanding of the cause-effect factors that lie behind the body's unique language. Foremost in specialized research have been Hans Selye, Spurgeon English, Johannes Weiss, Jerome Frank, E. Weaver Johnson, Roy Grinker, Franz Alexander, Milton Erickson, Karl Menninger, James Lynch, A. T. W. Simeons, Viktor Frankl, Lawrence LeShan and James A. Knight. To detail the nature and importance of their contributions would call for a library. Each in a unique and characteristic way has enriched the literature of psychosomatics and psychogenics.

The cumulative effect of research has slowly reduced the opposition of organized medicine to the claims of those who pay attention to more and more of the human response to life. A report presented at the 105th Annual Meeting of the American Medical Association[7] recognized the work of two physicians, Lawrence E. Hinkle, Jr and Harold G. Wolff, from the study programme of Human Health and Ecology of Man, working with two dozen colleagues in medicine, neurology, psychiatry, psychology, sociology and cultural anthropology, who affirmed that there is a clear parallel between disturbances of mood, thought and behaviour on the one hand and bodily illnesses on the other. They said there is no reason for believing that some diseases are psychosomatic while others are not, for they could find no aspect of the body system which isn't influenced by the brain's efforts to adapt, and that bodily processes changed by mental activity may lead to serious physical damage. In effect they were saying that all illness is psychosomatic, for the mind and the body are bound together like two sides of a zipper.

A group of researchers in and around Boston working in Massachusetts General Hospital, and in the universities of Harvard, Tufts and Brandeis have arrived at some theories about the onset of illness. They find that illness produces its presenting symptoms usually following some major emotional crisis in the life of the patient.[8] Erich Lindemann found that the elapsed time between acute grief and the onset of ulcerative colitis, tended to be about six months.[9] For asthma the onset might be but a few hours.[10] The development of the Epstein-Barr virus into mononeucliosis takes but a short while but the development of the same virus into lymphatic leukaemia calls for a chronic state of much longer duration.[11] The correlation of the onset of illness with a response to emotional crisis puts illness in a different category from that of usual diagnostic practices.

For years cancer was considered to be the one ailment that was not amenable to emotional causes. Now it appears to be one of the human maladies that is easily identified with acute or accumulated emotional stress.

Early in psychosomatic research, findings were reported that showed a relationship between tumours and emotions. Dunbar writes: 'Endocrine-hormonal system is among the

79

most responsive of all body systems to emotional stress . . . paranoid and cyclothymic groups are more susceptible to circulatory disorders and tumours . . . early diagnosis is aided by an evaluation of a personality profile . . . the personality history and character traits of patients suffering from cancer bore a relationship to prognosis . . . carcinogens are rarely specific: they simply set the stage for that variety of carcinoma to which a given organ is particularly susceptible . . . It is the accumulation of trifles rather than major traumatic events that produces serious dysfunction in the personality.'[12] 'Reports in the literature of malignant and non-malignant growths that disappear after psychotherapy in patients for whom the original diagnosis was adequately confirmed by specialists in the field . . . some cancers seem to be primarily a psychogenic syndrome occurring chiefly in menopausal women who suffer from emotional conflict, sexual maladjustment and frequent cancerophobia.'[13]

What Dunbar reported years ago has been elaborated by Dr Lawrence LeShan who has spent more than three decades studying and treating patients suffering with neoplastic tissue developments. He analyses with an in-depth counselling process the emotional profile of the patient, identifies the possible causitive agents and then works psychotherapeutically to help the patient modify the content of emotional life. His research on 'Spontaneous regressions' is verified by the retreat of cancers apparently due to changes in the patient's self-assessment and the generating of coping skills that may be employed in reorienting body chemistry and immunological resources. In a recent book he not only describes his research findings with a cohort of seventy-one cancer patients but he also shows the way changes to emotional states can modify the chemistry of the body.[14]

In conversation LeShan described how these changes can come about. Emotions affect the glandular system most immediately. The glands are the chemical factories of the body. The chemical resources of the body provide the immunity that resists viruses and other body intruders. The evidence seems to be that abnormal cell division is also controlled by the immune resources of the body which rejects what is not valid or acceptable. Perhaps hundreds of times a day abnormal cell division is stopped by the body's immune resources. But when chronic emotional stress causes the glands to function abnormally, the homeostatic balance is impaired and the body's normal chemical responses do not function adequately. So viral growth or abnormal cell division tend to be out of control. Viruses that are a constant in the body, like Epstein-Barr, are given a chance to develop with their damaging impact on the total organism. Thus the dynamics of some types of cancer are beginning to be more fully understood.

Medical practice generally uses assaultive techniques to slow up or eradicate the growth of abnormal cells. Chemotherapy assaults the unprogrammed cells that can do nothing but grow rapidly by feeding them a diet of poison with the intention that the healthy programmed cells will have strength to survive while the greedy abnormal cells will move towards gluttonous death. In other circumstances where the abnormal cells are growing in body parts that are not vital, the growth can be excised by surgery. At other times the cell growth can be retarded or eradicated by doses of radiation that burn out the weaker cancer cells while allowing the healthier normal cells to survive. Each of these assaultive methods takes its toll on the body.

Newer approaches have been developed that work within the body to stimulate immunological resources of the body to fight neoplastic tissue growth. Methods of aiding the body's immune resources with chemical boosters are an added method now being employed. Also experimentation is being done with energy therapy where the energy resources of the body are supplemented electronically or psychically. Psychotherapy which reduces stress and improves coping skills by changing self-image, life-styles and goals also seems to effectively change the ability of the body to resist illness and disease.

Research from within the medical community is challenging the nine basic assumptions that have been the foundation stones of biomedical practice. The understanding of other forces at work to produce the causes of morbid states of being are making it increasingly impossible to ignore the findings of psychosomatic research.

Speaking recently to a medical audience, Jonas Salk, co-developer of the polio vaccine, said that we are entering a new epoch in which holistic medicine will be the dominant model. 'We must use the biological paradigm to explore that level of complexity that we call the mind or spirit . . . being, ego and the phenomenon we refer to as transcendence or creation.' Defining further the new epoch, he said, 'I think of holism in its philosophical sense – the theory that whole entities are fundamental components of reality not just the sum of their parts . . . We need to adjust to this new reality, to adapt to it.'[15]

This new reality is built on two major components, energy physics and humanistic psychology as spiritual humanism. As one of the newer branches of psychological study it is based on the assumption that whatever is related to human experience is a proper focus for scientific study. The former assumption reflected in the nine points mentioned at the beginning of this chapter, that all experience could be divided into the subjective and the objective and that science was only interested in the latter, is no longer tenable. The whole of human experience has its unique validity.

As a charter member of the Academy of Parapsychology and Medicine, I have been able to watch through the years the accumulating evidence that we do not develop an understanding of persons and their problems by limiting the life phenomena that we will deign to study. Quite the opposite is being proved, for the more we explore the total experiences of human beings, the more we perceive about the vital forces that are actively interrelated. Speaking at a APM conference, Roy Menninger, head of the Menninger Foundation, said, 'The traditional ideas about medicine and the new concepts of man are on a collision course . . . We know now that health isn't just the absence of symptoms . . . We must have courage. We must recapture the person as the focus, or medicine will continue to sink in prestige.'[16] The reality of the person will not be perceived through a limited scientific study but rather from all the combined insights of science, philosophy and religion.

Interestingly, during the same period that medical science became restless with its own philosophical inadequacy, the world of the physical sciences was in a state of philosophical revolution. At the turn of the century physicists with a great sense of self-confidence were saying that there were just a few more missing pieces of the basic elements of creation and that when these were found the great mysteries would be finally explained. Humankind would then finally achieve mastery of the realm of material things. Then came Madame Curie and the door of energy physics was pushed ajar. Following in rapid succession came Nils Bohr, Albert Einstein, A. S. Eddington, Henry Margenau, Werner Heisenberg, Erwin Shrodinger, Aldous Huxley, Max Planck, Enrico Fermi, Wolfgang Pauli, J. Robert Oppenheimer and a host of other scientists who with their theoretical formulae and technical mastery changed our way of looking at life and the universe around us.

Not only was the concept of the law and order of the universe rapidly expanded but the role of material as the ultimately real gave place to energy forms as the basic form of ultimate reality. The implications were far-reaching. When the first atom bomb exploded in New Mexico in 1945 it spelled the end of dialectical materialism as a viable philosophy, and the

83

base of the communist political system was severely shaken. Religion that has tried to adapt and adjust to materialism was ill-prepared for the readjustments that came with a return to the purely spiritual reality base. Buildings, budgets and materialistically-oriented programmes had to be re-examined in the light of scientific mysticism. Education that had been teaching Newtonian physics with its materialistic and space-time orientation struggled to find something teachable amidst the immeasurable and imponderable concepts that moved beyond space and time and thought in terms of the infinitesimal and the timeless hidden in the fourth, fifth and sixth dimensions. Old measurements and old concepts became the illusory responses of limited sensory capacities. The ultimately real not only would not be responsive to our crude sensory equipment but it never could be. Even if we developed visual aids to see more clearly, by the time we had seen a particle that had a life span of a millionth of a second it would be long gone. The President of the Massachusetts Institute of Technology told a graduating class that the universe now appeared to be more like a great thought than a great thing. He also warned that knowledge is mushrooming so rapidly in the technical field that they were invited to return in eight years to have their brains retooled.

The world is changing so rapidly that ways of thinking are quickly outmoded. Familiar ways of believing are also proved to be inadequate. Approaches to healing and health are especially affected by burgeoning research and changes in philosophical assumptions about the nature of human beings and the nature of the universe itself. Our psychology is far more inclusive of human experience, and our cosmology is far less centred about material concepts and more resonant to energy processes than was the case just a few decades ago. Old ways of organizing knowledge have been outgrown. The systems view of humans, their world and their health becomes a new way of organizing our understanding and our concern about basic problems of life. Let us now explore what a systems approach to health can do to help resolve conflicts and release the insight, skills and energies that can be used to create new possibilities for healthful living.

9

New Partnerships

So far in our journey of exploration into the realm of health and illness we have tried to do several things. We have looked at personal responsibility for health and the role in the process of the person being healed. We have emphasized the unique and significant power of consciousness as a resource for a systems approach to healing. We have seen how consciousness is able to bring together, in a working unity, forces that in their more trivial uses would be divisive and might even cause illness.

Also we have been able to look at some of the unfortunate by-products of the mini-systems that have too often in the past worked against each other with human beings the ultimate losers. We now should be in a position to look beyond reductionism which seeks a simplistic answer to the problems of illness and health. When we are working with living systems we are dealing with process, not substance. When we say the whole is more than the sum of its parts we are not talking mathematics, but rather are focussing on the processes of collective behaviour that create new circumstances, new possibilities and new resources. There are no phenomena of life that are not molecular just as there is none that is only molecular.

Systems theory, we have argued, is basic to the understanding of life processes. We move beyond reductionism when we accept the idea that 'the system concept is the embodiment of the experience that there are patterned processes which owe their typical configuration not to a prearranged, absolutely sterotyped mosaic of single tracked component performances, but on the contrary, to the fact that the component activities have many degrees of freedom, but submit to the ordering restraints exerted upon them by the integral activity of the "whole" in its patterned systems dynamic'.[1]

The model of molecular biology tends to stop the action of living by creating models of molecules, for example, but molecules cannot be reduced to lifeless pictures or laboratory constructs. Efforts to do so produce only symbols, perhaps useful in teaching but far from life itself. Life cannot be atomized. It can be organized into systems that focus on the something more that life adds to matter. Just as the life of a city is more than the list of names in a telephone directory, and language is more than an alphabet, so a living system moves beyond reductionism. When mini-systems encounter life, life always finds the flaw in the mini-system. So homeostasis and intropsychic balance are systems approaches to the fact of life and make their claims based on the dynamics of the whole rather than the claims of unpredictable molecular action.

What is true of reductionism is certainly true of the philosophies often employed by reductionists. Mechanism tries to reduce all reality to mechanical process. While the human body employs some remarkable mechanisms of muscle and bone, it would be unrealistic to limit a human being to the mechanical processes so wisely employed. While a mechanical process is employed in walking, the process of walking is controlled by purpose as well as method – a 'where' as well as a 'how'.

The material perception of the human being adds a dimension to the merely mechanical, but still falls short. To assume that the body is only a complicated chemical factory with constant adjustment to environment and other conditioning factors fails to account for the fact that body chemistry responds to attitudes of mind and stimulation of emotions. More materialist systems would even deny the role of feelings as if they were inappropriate manifestations of the life process.

But vetoing the emotions does not seem to eliminate their effectiveness in modifying the materialistic systems that have been used to explain life and health. While the first three realities that deal with the physical and material are important in the total picture, we must also recognize that life is more than chemistry, and health is more than chemical balance inside of our skin.

One of the skills of those who depend on mini-systems is their ability to employ denial when confronted with facts or feelings that do not fit easily into their limited perspective. This has been implicit in the response of molecular biologists and biomedical practitioners when confronted with the research in psychosomatics. Denial is usually a primary defence against discomfort or hazardous growth. Gottleib Leibnitz (1654–1717) long ago observed that people tend to be right in their affirmations but wrong in their denials. The reason for this was that in their affirmations they were usually speaking from personal experience, where in their denial they were usually trying to discount the experience of others.[2] This may be why the mystical experience has been rejected in sweeping forms of denial. In psychotherapy the role of denial is clearly seen. 'Because denial must ignore data presenting themselves to the perceptory system and garnered by the memory apparatus, such a defence can operate only in the under-developed, infantile psyche, or in persons whose ego is weak or disturbed.'[3] People who find their mental and emotional security in mini-systems will use powerful emotional investments to protect themselves. This leads to rejection of truth and further retreat into the limiting and limited mini-systems.

In the face of the burden of consciousness and the demands that it places on life for discipline and action, it is easy to understand why so often there has been a retreat to reductionism, mechanism, materialism and denial. These forms of response to mind-stretching truth are self-destructive and may lead to frustration, depression and group paranoia. We deserve something better, especially when so many persons are affected by health care modalities.

Perhaps we are socially and scientifically ready for a major change of mood. Instead of using mini-systems to escape from responsibility we may be ready to adopt a systems approach that can bring together our best insights in a mood of shared exploration and mutual responsibility. In order to achieve this goal we need larger loyalties and more effective partnerships among those who are concerned about health. Not only is there a need for individual discipline, but also a new concept of the disciplined team. Such a field is emerging in scientific research. Most of the important developments of our day are not the result of an isolated Edison working late in his laboratory. Rather, we find teams of scientists working together and communicating creatively across national boundaries and scientific specializations. We have new relationships unknown a few decades ago. Biochemistry, astro-physics, astrobiology and radiation chemistry and many more coupled specializations have adventured across new frontiers to new shared insights. Certainly the incentives exist for bringing together in a similar manner the disciplines that could influence illness and health.

New partnership and disciplined team work can strengthen the belief in the value of a specialization along with a strong conviction that through sharing there can be important benefits for all concerned. Shared concerns also call for shared responsibilities. Recently a request came in from a midwestern clinic that wanted to practise holistic medicine. They wanted to find a clergyman who believed as vigorously in his special discipline as the physicians believed in theirs. The request carried the information that they had already interviewed nearly two dozen chaplains and had not found one who believed in the spiritual power that contributed to healing as much as the physicians believed in the efficacy of their own training and resources. They commented further that most of the chaplains had been trained in hospitals and had been so imbued with the medical model that they had lost sight of or rejected the special resource they could bring to the healing team.

Shared concerns calls for a melding of skills, abilities for communication and a tolerance for differing perspectives. There must be a body of knowledge and experience that each brings to the team. There must also be a personal discipline that bears fruit in the belief in the contribution each specialization can make. Also there must be a mutual respect and openness of communication that makes possible shared insights and methods of intervention. In the past this opportunity for genuine sharing has been limited by language specialization for it is difficult to talk with those who are unable to share a professional vocabulary. Free communication also involves truth and this has not always been present among professional groups where sibling rivalry may linger on. Such difficulties place limits on fruitful partnerships. Many times late at night in conferences or retreats, physicians, psychologists and pastors had talked with refreshing openness. Such sessions lead to professional growth as well as personal healing. The doubts and fears and even loneliness that weigh heavily on life among professionals have been dissipated and almost always the sessions have ended with the expressed feeling, 'We should do this more often.'

I experienced a postgraduate course in health care and team work when each morning for more than a year the chief of medicine, the chief of surgery, the chief of psychiatry and the chief of chaplains sat down with the sick calls of the day. In the scope of a few minutes the particulars of each case were explored and recommendation for intervention suggested. In mutual respect each member of the team was heard and before the staff meeting ended individual or shared responsibility was assumed for each patient. Also in the psychiatric clinic that I headed the staff meeting each Monday morning brought the twenty staff persons together to talk about cases and explore modes of treatment that might be recommended. The pool of resources was dipped into according to the needs of the individual patient and the shared insight of the professional team.

Already in many institutions a philosophy of patient care is emerging that considers needs in a broader perspective. The psychologist and the social worker as well as physiotherapists and other counsellors are recognized for what they have to contribute to patient welfare. The time seems ripe for us to add yet another modification to the process by changing the heirarchical structure and creating a value system based on what the team member can offer to patient care rather than personal status in the treatment centre pecking order.

This is the point where the unique contribution of holistic medicine may provide an organizing point. With its basic loyalty to a maxi-system approach to human health needs, the loyalties could be centred in the person who is ill rather than in the professional loyalties of the traditional providers of health care. Then the nurse, the psychologist, the chaplain and the physician could talk, work and serve as equals. As we pointed out earlier in this exploration, one of the main reasons the insights of psychosomatic medical research have been ignored is that the physician does not have the time to employ its insights as practice is now organized. So physicians tend to retreat to the time-economical methods of chemical and surgical intervention. With a competent, trustworthy and dependable team the work can be shared and each member of the team can not only do what they can do best but they can share insights so that the patient can benefit from more understanding and more widely employed skills. This is a method made to order for the philosophy and practice of holistic medicine.

Yet holistic medicine is not just a matter of bringing together a team of people who trust one another and share their skills. The new understanding of the role of the patient makes an active participation possible by the person who moves from passive to active in health care. In chapter 12 (pp. 123f.) we shall note Dr Harry Lipscomb's experience monitoring the physical responses of the astronauts in outer space and its impact on medical practice. What has happened under less dramatic circumstances could become a part of practice generally. Under professional guidance the power and vital resources of the patient might be set free to add significantly to the therapeutic process.

As we noted earlier, it is now quite common for people to take an active interest in their health through preventive measures such as wise nutrition, sound exercise, relaxation, concern about genetic weakness and modified life-styles. Also in the preventive category are the campaigns against health hazards implicit in smoking, eating additive-laden food, and over-dependence on drugs.

Holistic approaches to health would learn the special skills necessary to translate the language of the body into healthful understanding of body needs. The metaphors of the body are constantly sending messages that can be understood by those who know the special code of the body. No one has ever seen a toothache but when a tooth begins to ache it does not call for special training to know that the tooth is telling us that something is wrong with the tooth. Some metaphors are not that explicit and require special skills from the translator. If we are concerned with more than symptom management we will want to listen in depth to the messages the body sends us. In the long run the proper understanding of the ailment and its unique body language becomes a significant part of the prevention or recurrence. It can lead to a modification of a life-style which, left unmodified, might cause more serious illness were the body signals ignored.

It has been observed that there is a cumulative effect in illness that results from ignoring body metaphors. A large number of common colds tend to weaken body resources and trigger more serious maladies. Pneumonia strikes more than twice in the same place. When the warning signs of the Epstein-Barr virus at work in mononucleosis are ignored, that same virus, Epstein-Barr, may move from its benign form to its malignant manifestation in lymphatic leukaemia.[4] One of the major opportunities afforded by the holistic approach to illness is the multiprofessional approach to the language of the body as differing skills are employed in listening to what the body is saying by its illness.

At Walter Reed Hospital where I have served on the staff, there has been instituted a professorship of holistic medicine. One of its functions is to supervise a wellness clinic. Here patients are not only able to terminate their treatment for past illness but are given training in avoiding future illness. They are encouraged to take more responsibility for their own health. They are encouraged to avoid the things that made them sick in the past and learn new ways of managing their personal and social life so that they will not develop the kinds of stress that made them ill.

The role of the professor of holistic medicine is shown by this illustration. In addition to teaching he provides an alternative treatment modality. An officer who had served in Vietnam had responsibility for sending men on patrol and into combat. Many men did not come back. The officer years later complained of pains in his back growing increasingly severe. These painful spasms became so excruciating that he was hardly able to bear them. He was willing to endure almost anything to get relief. A medical consultation decided that major surgery was indicated to relieve the intense pain. The day before the surgery was scheduled the professor of holistic medicine visited the officer and talked with him about the pain and asked when it had begun. It appeared that it began when the officer felt deep guilt for the death of men he sent into combat. The more he talked about the matter the more feelings he expressed. An accumulation of long denied emotion came

93

pouring out. It was observed that after this session of emotional outpouring, the pain subsided. The professor of holistic medicine asked the surgeon if he would be able to postpone the operation until the professor could have a few more sessions with the officer and his deeply repressed feelings of guilt. The request was granted. The end result was that after several more sessions of actively coping with the powerful feelings of guilt there was a relaxation of stress and the mediating of the healing insight that changed the inner tensions and the spasticities of the officer's body, mind and spirit. The surgery was finally cancelled as unnecessary for the relief from pain came about by the use of an alternative form of healing intervention.

This illustration shows what is possible under some circumstances. But it is only possible when trust and co-operation are at work on the healing team. At several points in the process communication might have broken down. Hurt feelings or injured pride as well as prejudice might have prevented a desirable outcome and the patient would have been the loser. We may have arrived at the place where what happens to the patient will be examined from a broader perspective growing from mutual trust, increased understanding of psychodynamics and the willingness to give the team approach necessary for holistic health practice a chance to show its possibilities. The stage seems set, and certainly the time is propitious for this step to be taken.

10

New Practices

When a new social and scientific climate emerges, forms of response begin to develop. At first the changes may be almost imperceptible because modifications are so gradual. Some pioneering spirits more adventurous than others started to react to the research in psychosomatics with a clearly directed purpose. During the fifties the Laymans Movement held a series of seminars which brought together leading figures in orthodox medicine along with others who were using alternative modes of healing. Having been a part of these seminars and being intrigued by the type of issues that were discussed I have treasured the transcribed reports of these conferences as frontier points towards holistic goals in the healing process. With great care and openness the physicians examined in depth unorthodox healers Olga and Ambrose Worrall, Dora VanGelder, Agnes Sanford and others who had been leaders in exploring some alternate ways of treating illness and disease. There were moments of tension when basic assumptions were challenged as different understandings of human beings and their health were openly confronted.

At one of the Wainright House sessions this open confrontation was met directly. A learned Jesuit who apparently felt threatened by my efforts to explain paranormal approaches to healing spoke up and said quite bluntly, 'I think you are a fake and a fraud. To put it simply, I think you are a phoney'. Having always felt that a defensive position has an inherent weakness, I said nothing. Dr Lawrence LeShan, well known for his support for alternative programmes for cancer treatment, was serving as chairman of the session. Addressing the Jesuit priest, Dr LeShan said: 'I know you have bursitis in your right shoulder so severe that you have had to give up your favourite game of tennis. Suppose we let Edgar work on it?' After a few minutes of discussion in which the Jesuit priest took a strong negative attitude, it was decided to try a form of intervention that employed prayer and the laying on of hands. The priest was asked to show the group the limits that the bursitis placed on arm mobility. He could not comb his hair or lift a spoon higher than his mouth, and even then with a rather contorted movement. First I asked the group, which seemed highly interested in the proceedings, if they would join with me in the attitude of prayer surrounding both of us in loving concern. Then after clearing my mind and bringing my thoughts into sharp focus I moved into an altered state of consciousness. Placing one hand on the priest's shoulder just above the joint, and the other just below it at the armpit, I remained in silence and deep concentration for several minutes. After a while I suggested to the priest that he slowly raise his arm, doing so gently to avoid any discomfort. As he raised his arm higher and higher members of the group sitting about the room said that the joint emitted snapping and cracking sounds like a famous breakfast cereal. Before long the priest jumped from his chair and started swinging his arm as if he were making mighty serves on the tennis court. Incidentally he came to me in private and said he was sorry that he had called me a 'phoney' but that with his precise training in logic it seemed reasonable to reject phenomena that didn't fit a logical framework and that you have to experience some things before you extended your logical framework. The important fact, however, was that this was done in the presence of a number of people who knew well the perspectives of bio-medical practice but were willing to confront something that demanded a re-examination of their former limits of thought and practice. Even within the most orthodox of traditions there is a new willingness to confront new ways of looking at life and health.

Perhaps one of the best illustrations of this mood of openness was Cancer Dialogue '80, A Multidimensional approach. Called An International Symposium of Physicians, Scientists and Researchers, it met for four days in New York during October 1980. Eighteen research physicians and nine other persons as varied as Linus Pauling and Pir Vilayat, Lawrence LeShan with his experience in understanding the dynamics of spontaneous regressions to Guy Newell from Anderson Hospital and Tumour Institute in Texas, all concerned about the limits of their knowledge, were ready and willing to learn of one another. As during the International Year of the Child and the Geophysical Year old boundaries were erased in a common concern for a great human necessity.

Not only is there a change in the methods of co-operation and confrontation in healing, but there are developing conflicting ideas of responsibility. Two basic positions are considered. One centres on personal responsibility, as if health were a personal matter. Another approach thinks of health in special terms. Many programmes that have been effective in controlling disease have been clearly social such as the use of quarantine and isolation with communicable diseases, as well as massive programmes of vaccination and immunization against the spread of contagious disease. It has been estimated that with health insurance, medicare and medicaid a major portion of expense for health care is now spread through society by various forms of social responsibility. One of the major political questions now has to do with the limits of social responsibility in the area of health care. This is further complicated by debates on the conflict of personal and social responsibility. Dr Ronald Glasser, Professor at the Medical School of the University of Minnesota, asserts that cigarette smoking is the major health problem of today, causing three hundred and sixty thousand deaths a year in the USA alone.

The Hastings Report raises the question concerning who should bear the burden of those who suffer the consequences of their own anti-health activities. Should non-smokers carry the economic burden for those who refuse to heed warnings and add to product costs by lost days of employment and lengthy forms of illness with hospital costs and heavy drains upon the health care resources?[1]

One of the objections to the emphasis on holistic healing is that it provides benefits to an elite group who have the time and the skills to use mental power for health purposes. The mass of people who live at a less privileged status in society may not have accessible the disciplines and intellectual understanding that are basic to the mode of intervention holistic methods require. Is holistic healing to be used as a device to escape social responsibility for the easing of the suffering of those who do not have the resources for taking personal responsibility in health matters? We have long known that those who live a deprived existence are more apt to retreat into forms of drug dependence as a way of easing boredom and emotional stress. The use of the more prevalent addictive drugs such as nicotine and alcohol provide the mild relief and escape from the burdens born by the emotionally over-wrought, the impoverished and underprivileged. Would the growing emphasis on the resources of holistic medicine create a larger gap between the privileged and underprivileged? Would the concept of personal responsibility reduce the appeal of social programmes to provide the health care that is essential for the socially deprived? While this could be a tendency if the alternatives were unexamined, it would certainly not find its final expression in an either-or approach. Here again a larger perspective would use all of the resources for health and properly gear them to the existent social needs. So it would not be merely an awareness of the problems, but would lift social concern to a higher order of response in social responsibility.

build the inner resources that could stabilize life and produce a more adequate person for future living.

Clergypersons would enhance their role on the healing team by developing a greater understanding of the needs of the sick. The metaphoric language of the body might first be interpreted by them before the symptoms became disabling. While this might be an understanding of the language of the body quite different from that of the biomedical specialist, it could supplement it in meeting the needs of the patient. The superficial retreat into magic and denial has long been a part of the religious scene. Instead of developing coping skills the religious community has often encouraged people to sing lustily 'God will take care of you', or to assume that Jesus 'all my sins and griefs will bear'. The superficial retreat into magic which involves a distortion of reality encourages retreat from reality and should be studiously avoided. Rather than working against each other, if the spiritual counsellor and biomedical practitioner were to consult frequently, this would make it possible for extra resources within the patient and the healing team to be activated. Instead of diverting energy into escapes from responsibility the partnership between patient and members of the healing team would be strengthened. In this type of shared activity all concerned could nourish the growing edge of their patient's understanding and so enhance the usefulness of their intervention.

The religious organization could embody many of the activities of the healing team. Having been a member of the national advisory committee of Hospice, Inc., from its beginning, I have been aware of the role that trained and dedicated volunteers, largely recruited from the churches, have been able to perform. In order to aid families who wanted to provide patient care in the home setting during the final days of life, when the facilities of the home were limited, the skilled workers from Hospice, Inc. could come in to give relief in patient care, needed rest to the family and also guidance in ways of meeting aspects of the crisis that were unfamiliar.

At other times the clergy could perform ministries that were not so much a matter of dealing with illness as they were with being close enough to people to perceive the initial signs of trouble and intercede when the intervention might do the most good. The pastoral person is often the only professional in the community who has ready access to the homes of people. So the pastoral person has the rights and privileges of the caring shepherd. This makes it possible to observe people in many life situations and by paying careful attention the pastor may be sensitive to problems as they develop and often before they become critical. By keeping a close watch for relevant information concerning people in the parish, the pastor may serve as an outpost for the professional team and alert other members of the team so that wise intervention may occur.

This alertness could make it possible for a valued counsellor to be readily available to provide aid and counsel when it is most needed, at the time of the initial shock of an emotional crisis.[3]Further it would change the goal of the counsellor, for instead of seeking to help the person adapt and adjust to the crisis in terms of passive acceptance, the effort would be made to assist him or her to accept an active role and direct the inner power towards positive goals. Often in crises people think they have no alternatives and that they must be compliant and accepting. Now it is becoming increasingly clear that the positive alternatives are not only possible but highly preferable. The patient can be a part of the solution as well as a part of the problem. The goal of counselling as well as the role of the counsellor can be quite different when they are all part of the healing team.

As Viktor Frankl has pointed out, the counsellor, when entering into an encounter with a patient, cannot help but reveal or reflect the philosophy which is basic to the mode of intervention.[4] Dr Frankl says that in reality the doctor cannot long remain in an aloof and protected position of the disinterested physician seeing only a portion of the total person. So the physician who thinks about the deeper human needs of the patient inevitably takes on some of the role of the minister.

The counsellor, whether religious, biomedical or psychological is engaged with the patient in determining acceptable alternatives. Will it be breakdown, breakup or breakthrough? In the breakdown the patient is apt to be following the mechanical model where the physical item can bear only so much stress before the weight of events fractures the resources of the patient. Then the model of the machine suggests collapse and replacement.

Also there can be the psychological model of giving up in the face of what appears to be intolerable stress. The breakup can show in human relations. In marriage the breakup often occurs when the people involved decide that they do not have the resources or the inclination to confront a problem in terms of the potential for solution. They give up and break up with all of the attendant complications for usually such action creates more problems than it resolves. The breakup may also be in an attitude that relates to illness, for a person may direct resources towards a goal until some careless word or attitude destroys resolve and determination and the patient gives up in the face of pain and the unacceptable life-style that illness imposes. So they may retreat from resolve and actively or tacitly say to themselves that the struggle for health is not worth the effort it requires, and in their personal battle capitulate to their illness. So often in working with the catastrophically ill persons the critical moment may come when a thoughtless word or act undermines personal resolve and the patient is defeated by the process of disease.[5]

In contrast to breakdown as a mechanical model or breakup from psychological resolve there is the possibility for breakthrough to the discovery of new powers, new resources and new skills that may emerge from the team approach to a sick person. Often it may involve a subtle balance of internal resources for managing life and its stresses. A young man suffering from virulent illness was judged by the medical staff to be dying and without the vital resource to survive the next night. During the evening a message came to the chaplain on duty stating that the patient's wife had died due to an overdose of drugs. Knowing the circumstances of the young man's life the chaplain felt he should make every effort to deliver the message. The young man had been in unresolved conflict between his straight, conservative parents and his wife who was a member of the counterculture. He was caught in the breach between the intransigence of his parents and the inability and disinclinations of his wife to make major changes in her life-style. The tension centred in the conflict of loyalties within the catastrophically ill patient. The chaplain checked with the physician who said the patient was in a coma and probably not able to respond. However, the chaplain felt it was his duty to try. Getting as close as possible to the patient's ear he enunciated the message as clearly as possible, repeating it several times. There was no response from the patient. However, next morning the patient was better. The release from the deep inner conflict appeared to have affected body chemistry enough to tip the balance homeostatically. Over a period of several weeks there was slow improvement and in a few weeks time the patient was able to leave the hospital. Intropsychic balance and modified homeostatic balance are so closely bound together that cause-effect processes may become obscured. Even tragic news may be organized by the deeper levels of consciousness to relieve life-destroying emotional stress. The inclination to break down or give up can move towards a breakthrough when the healing team refuses to limit its efforts to the negative alternatives.

Dramatic new phenomena in health care are being developed from within biomedical practice and the ancillary professions concerned about health care. While problems of adaptation and adjustment persist, the rewards of team work and co-operation seem to be worth the effort to continue the exploration. New ways of working together may reveal powers within waiting to be organized and directed by those who have the wisdom and courage to believe in it.

11

New Research and New Skills

The last hundred years, with their burgeoning activity in the personality sciences, have produced much insight that broadens our perspectives in the healing arts. Things that at one time might have been considered irrelevant are now recognized as having considerable importance to matters of health and wholeness. Ancient wisdom that has been considered long outmoded may now be seen as basically sound. Even old wives' tales that were ridiculed are now seen as containing the accumulated wisdom of the long eons of human experience.

For instance for years it was assumed that our knowledge of prenatal development superseded the old wives' tales about maternal influence on the unborn. However, the tragic experience with thalidomide showed that deforming chemicals were able to pass through the membranes that surround zygote, embryo and foetus. This started a whole new type of research and the results have been startling. Now it is known that the number of stillbirths among women who smoke during pregnancy is much higher than among women who do not smoke. The reason appears to be in the specialized nature of the tissues of the placenta which are programmed for their special nine-month function. When the minute muscle tissues are expanded and contracted excessively in response to the chemical effect of the nicotine, their resiliancy is used up in eight months with a consequent inability to support life through the normal term of the pregnancy. Similar research of the Sudden Infant Crib Death organization indicates that the death rate from this mysterious ailment is twice as high among children whose mothers smoked during pregnancy. With hard drug usage by the mother, babies may be born already addicted. The drug experience unquestionably damages the physical equipment of the neonate. Such research makes it quite clear that responsibility is a more complicated and far-reaching influence on health than has been assumed. What was at one time considered to be merely a matter of taste and human freedom is now quite obviously a significant matter of moral responsibility affecting life and death.

Some of the research that has important bearing on health and holistic processes at first appears to have little relevance. Dr Lawrence Abt, a projective psychologist, had the feeling that there were significant social factors that provided thera-peutic intervention with many types of human stress. He set out to find what they might be. He was aware of the fact that every culture had a well-structured form of ritualized behav-iour that was more or less taken for granted. Dr Abt felt this group behaviour might be more important than most people realized. So he went to work to explore rites, rituals and ceremonies to see what they contributed to health. In his book, *Acting Out*,[1] he shows how these forms of group behaviour provide a language of the emotions that is direct and specific and does not need to be channelled through intellectualizing processes. These forms of direct behaviour make it possible to direct consciousness with physical co-operation, for the large muscle system is engaged. Similarly the glandular system is used, for basic to all acting-out behaviour is the direct access to the emotions, and the emotions most immediately affect the glandular system. Also group acceptance and support may directly take the place of intellectualisms which become unnecessary, for everyone knows what is going on and why. Understanding follows without interpretation, because these types of group behaviour are socially-oriented, with the group support being implicit. Dr Abt considers that these rights, rituals and ceremonies are a community resource providing the first line of defence against the type of stress that could over-tax the coping skills and lead to illness.

Dr Abt further found in his study that every culture seems to provide those acting-out procedures in ways that are appropriate for meeting the stress that comes with major life crises. So he finds these forms of group behaviour at the time of birth, onset of adolescence, marriage, and times of political, social or historical importance. Also at times of illness and death ceremonial acting-out has importance. An interesting chapter in Dr Abt's book is entitled 'Acting In'. It points out what happens when persons are denied by choice or circumstance the opportunity to act out feelings in socially valid ways. The powerful emotions that are related to stress points in life are then turned inward and detoured through other channels. These other channels may reduce the natural healthful processes of life, reduce immunity and lead to the development of infectious or neoplastic body conditions.

It would seem that on the basis of this and other similar research we could take a new look at the contribution to health that would be provided by stress-related social behaviour. Alvin Toffler has pointed out that one of the problems in a mobile culture like ours, where a quarter of the families move every year, is that social roots and the ceremonies that go with social rootage are severely interfered with.[2] The loss of roots can produce social instability with its effect on health. Some of the old ways of doing things need to be examined and replaced but the important thing seems to be that we need to restore the equivalent of what was lost. We have seen the political implications of this type of future shock where people in frenzied irrationality retreat into the mood of the past that is already gone rather than face the future whose problems must inevitably be resolved.

Holistic approaches to health would not ignore any of the personal and social resources available to help provide healthful attitudes and practices for life. Some healing activity is centred about forms of ritualized behaviour traditional in the church. There is evidence of its efficacy in reaching directly to life-disrupting emotional areas. For instance, a colleague who happens to be also a brother-in-law recounts a story from his own pastoral experience. On the day he was planning to get an early start on vacation with his wife, he received a call from a woman who said the physician had told them her mother was dying and could not survive another twenty-four hours. She further said her mother did not want to die without the sacrament of holy communion. With quite limited enthusiasm my colleague agreed to drive fifteen miles across Brooklyn on a hot summer day to administer the sacrament. He said he did it with a minimum of sufferance and time and hurried off on his delayed start of vacation. So it was quite a surprise a month later to return to his parish church and find this supposedly dying woman sitting on the front pew with her health restored. The essential element of this story, however, was that this woman who had been born and brought up in the Roman Catholic Church had been divorced and therefore excluded from the sacramental life of her church. When she became ill her deep concern was that she might die without the benefit of a final acceptance by the Christian church, at least sacramentally. The emotional relief from the sacramental act administered with limited enthusiasm appears to have been sufficient to meet the emotional needs of this patient and when she was prepared to die in peace she found that she was prepared to live in renewed health. The experience of this type of sacramental intervention is cumulative and quite convincing as a resource for healing. Catholic priests tell me that it is quite a common thing for parishioners to have a healing experience related to the administering of the final ceremonial act of the church. Emotional release that is verified and fortified by an authoritative person and institution seems to be able to speak directly to the deeper levels of the emotions with the basic change in body chemistry thereby induced. The restoration of health is an attested concommitant. Similarly the bedside manner of the physician mediating his authoritative type of healing intervention with accompanying tender love and care can often be equally efficacious.

In recent years, through the work of Dr Dolores Kreiger and Dr Frederick LeBoyer, a new appreciation of the value of therapeutic touch has been developed. Dr Kreiger is a professor at the school of nursing at New York Hospital. She teaches a popular course in the healing touch. Her rationale is that nurses touch more people in more places more often than anyone else on the healing team. Therefore how they do it becomes an important factor in assessing the results. In a recent lecture given in San Anselmo, California, where I shared the programme with her, she said that if a nurse is hurried, careless and hurting, the emotional response of the patient is expressed in a retarding of the healing process. Resentment, fear and distress have their negative impact on the glandular system with physically measurable results. Quite the opposite is true when the nurse is gentle, patient and concerned. The mediating of tender love and care may be measurable in a positive sense just as the opposite seems to be. The total being of the patient responds to loving touch and kindly words expressed along with it. This research and practice fortifies the idea of the laying on of hands and gives validity to employing of a cosmic dimension through the use of prayer which helps the patient preoccupied with the painful 'in there' to broaden the perspective on life in such a way that the resources 'out there' may be more readily accessible.

Dr Frederick LeBoyer, through his research and writing, has made it possible for many persons to have a better understanding of the importance of prenatal and neonatal touch. It is his idea that if the birth is an abrupt and painful break in organic experience it may set a pattern for life and create a never-ending series of crises rooted in the expectancy of pain and distress. However, he feels that the alternative is a valid

110

possibility. If the gentle massage that occurs when the foetus is immersed in the amniotic fluid can be reinstituted immediately after birth the neonate begins to adjust to the new environment with feelings of pleasant touch. If added to this there are gentle sounds, quiet music and the general atmosphere of loving concern the infant can early develop positive responses to life that may well set a pattern for all the rest of life. Then instead of having birth be a painful and isolating form of stress, it may well be the opposite with new life being experienced with joy and each new life event approached with anticipation.[3]

Approaches to health and wholeness have broad dimensions; the concern for the neonate on the one hand and the aged who have the benefits of Hospice, Inc. What we are seeing is a new perception of health not so much as absence of physical symptoms as enrichment of life through social interaction and a wide variety of meaningful forms of communication and relationship. This changes the focus of healthful considerations from biology to psychology and religion, from survival to meaning and purpose.

This broadened base for understanding health could make it possible for holistic teamwork to develop new concepts of the person, well beyond a preoccupation with mere symptoms, as the possibilities for becoming a super-healthy person become more important. Here we begin to move in the direction of concepts that may best be defined as being in the realm of mystical integration of all of life in terms of its most abundant possibilities.

Dr Peterim Sorokin of Harvard has developed the thesis that the genius is a person who knowingly or unknowingly possesses a rich psychic endowment that is constantly working for a higher form of integration within the individual. The psychic gifts of the genius personality make it possible to have instant knowledge where other persons must struggle with the more usual approaches to knowing.[4]

Dr Alexis Carrel, formerly medical director of the Rocke-feller Research Center, puts it more specifically. He writes:

Men of genius, in addition to their powers of observation and comprehension, possess other qualities such as intui-tion and creative imagination. Through intuition they learn things ignored by other men, they perceive relations be-tween seemingly unrelated phenomena, they unconscious-ly feel the presence of the unknown treasure. All great men of science have intuition, they know without analysis, with-out reasoning, what is important for them to know . . . This phenomenon, in former times, was called intuition . . . Certainty derived from science is very different from that derived from faith. The latter is more profound. It cannot be shaken by argument. It resembles the certainty given by clairvoyance. But, strange to say, it is not completely foreign to science. Obviously, great discoveries are not the product of intelligence alone.[5]

If the physical body is a manifestation of the quality of mind and spirit of the person inhabiting it, it would seem obvious that the higher the level of consciousness the nearer the person would come to being a super-healthy person. Long ago Martin Luther said, 'Heavy thoughts bring on physical maladies; when the soul is oppressed so is the body.' George Bernard Shaw expressed the inverse when he wrote, 'Mens sana in corpore sano is a foolish saying. The sound body is a product of a sound mind.' Yet both are probably in error if they think of the mind as the seat of intelligence rather than the conscious-ness as the centre for integrating the richness of body, mind and spirit. Nearly twenty-five centuries ago Plato saw this integrative relationship when he wrote: 'The cure of many diseases is unknown to the physicians of Hellas, because they are ignorant of the whole, which ought to be studied also: for the part can never be well unless the whole is well . . . This . . . is the great error of our day in the treatment of the human body, that the physicians separate the soul from the body.' If we are to discover the possibility of a superhealthy person we must move beyond negative assessment of the symptoms to the possible achievements of the whole person functioning at maximum potential.

The concept of the super-healthy person that may develop from our interest in the fuller potential of integrated body, mind and spirit, cannot be found through intellectual processes alone. Rather it will come through some integration of the total being which in the past has usually been referred to as revelation. Previously we have usually tried to make revelation something mysterious that comes to us from outside and beyond. Perhaps we are overlooking the fact that the greatest of revelations come from deep within where the higher consciousness, or the inner kingdom responds to the divine image seeking to free itself from our preoccupation with the material, the physical and the enslaving influence of our attachment to the artificial realities.

The idea of revelation is avoided by many because it moves beyond easy modes of thought. But within human nature there seem to be meeting places for elements of reality that are larger than the measuring sticks we would hold against them. This inclination to be afraid of what we cannot control by measurement seems to be deep seated in the emotions of people, even those who are devoted to contemporary scientific perspectives with its sense of indeterminacy, infinite and eternal. The measurement does not really do anything to anything. Everything remains the same except for the illusion of control.

The nature of the true revelation moves beyond human doubts to achieve the phenomena of self-realization and communication with a quality of relationship which Gerald Heard calls 'Higher Prayer'. The psychiatrist Richard Maurice Bucke experienced this revelation and called it 'cosmic consciousness'.[6] This phenomenon, quite rare in nature, appears as a form of illumination, where insight into the nature of reality and the function of consciousness is brought together in what had until then been kept apart by the influence of limited perceptions of reality. Barriers to perception are eliminated and with rare clarity of seeing, the being is fully aware that all is one and that one encompasses the perceiving being. It was in that state of being that George Washington Carver talked with peanuts and then listened, and there was revealed to him knowledge about the secret structure of matter upon which he was then able to reach in such a way that he was able to develop more than two hundred products from the lowly peanut and transform the economy of the south.[7]

Albert Einstein shared such an experience which he described in his little book *Cosmic Religion*. He writes:

The religious geniuses of all time have been distinguished by this cosmic religious sense, which recognizes no dogmas nor God made in man's image . . . How can this cosmic religious experience be communicated from man to man if it cannot lead to a definite conception of God or a theology? It seems to be the most important function of art and of science to arouse and keep alive this feeling in those who are receptive . . . Only those who have dedicated their lives to similar ends can have a living conception of the inspiration which gave those men the power to remain loyal to their purpose in spite of countless failures. It is the cosmic religious sense that grants this power. A contemporary has rightly said that the only deeply religious people of our largely materialistic age are the earnest men of research.[8]

From many sources we find confirmation of the idea that in science and in holistic approaches to health there are inviting frontiers to explore. Some of our areas of research have been constricted by the limits of the methods we employ and the philosophical base from which we move. Human beings have much more potential than we have credited to them. Super-healthy persons are a possibility. Let us push out the boundaries, free from the fears and prejudices that have constrained us in the past.

12

The Need to Accelerate

It is quite human to wonder about the future. Futurists make a profession of it. They look at what is happening in the present, feed their statistics into computers and predict what the end results of current trends may be. Let us play the futurist's game for a while as we look at trends in health care today.

The futurist starts with questions. What is the meaning of what we see happening today? Are the meanings clear or obscured? What will the present trends do to shape tomorrow? Is it possible to influence the trends so that we can avoid failure and catastrophe and achieve wiser and more creative possibilities in the days ahead?

Alvin Toffler has examined some of our current personal and social behaviour to try to understand what lies behind irrational forms of action. Why do we resist creative change and try to retreat to old and familiar ways of doing things? What have we lost in rapid change that impairs our perception in the present and prevents us from adopting more intelligent approaches to the future?

Let us confront some of these questions as we look at some areas of concern in assessing modern medical practice. What will be our health problems in the twenty-first century? What will we do about medical costs? Will medical practice become increasingly mechanized? What will be the future of specialization? How does computerization fit into the picture in terms of humanization or mechanization? What about some of the failures in medical practice?

Materialism is a philosophical theory which regards matter

116

and its motion as constituting the universe and all phenomena including those of mind as due to material agencies. Its prime devotion is to the material rather than the non-material, the emotional, the psychological or the spiritual.

The philosophical base for medical practice during the major portion of the last century has been basically materialistic. The material body has been central in establishing the causes of disease, the research relating to its management and the concept of the person who is diseased.

From the concepts of Frederick LeBoyer and his interest in the bonding of newborn babies (see above, pp. 110f.) to the influence of the Hospice movement with its concern about how people end their earthly pilgrimage and die, non-material considerations are exerting a renewed influence upon life and thought. This has a direct bearing on concepts of health and medical practice.

Morals and social practices also affect how people think of themselves. The rigid moral codes of Puritanism certainly had their bearing on emotional states that affected life. The mood of growing permissiveness and moral laxity may reduce some forms of stress but at the same time they will inevitably destroy the security systems that have been sustained by rigid codes of behaviour.

As we look at the problems of health care in the next century we will have to look at both the practical and theoretical matters that underlie our understanding of illness and health. In this chapter we will be exploring the more practical considerations that affect our ways of thinking and acting in health matters, and in the next chapter we will consider the theoretical implications that emerge from history and research.

One of the major considerations leading to a re-examination of health care problems is costs. Traditional forms of health care are rapidly pricing themselves out of the market. In a health centre in the USA where I serve on the board of directors one of our major problems is unpaid and uncollect-able bills. Changes in government policy affecting health care are only compounding the problem. People want health care but can't afford it. With intensive care and trauma units costing so much as one thousand dollars a day, and ordinary hospital beds two hundred dollars a day, a life's savings can be gobbled up in a few days. People are obliged to consider alternative ways of managing health problems. Either the state must move in with massive programmes of health care or the ill and diseased person must look elsewhere for release from physical distress.

What lies behind the high cost of health care? Basically there are three sources of increased costs: the cost of equipment, the cost of personnel and the cost of education.

The costs of equipment are basically building and mainten-ance, mechanical devices, electronic equipment and chemical resources.

Every city and town has experienced building programmes for hospitals with large outlays for material, labour and fund raising. The staff required to maintain old and new buildings becomes a constant which adds to the cost of every day of hospitalization.

I asked the medical director of a highly successful trauma unit how he could justify the costs of his unit. He responded that the helicopter alone was an investment that ran into hundreds of thousands of dollars, with specially trained personnel on duty one hundred and sixty-eight hours a week to maintain and operate it. Then he explained that the use of ambulances to rescue people in automobile accidents was proving to be increasingly difficult because of traffic problems in and around accident scenes. The helicopter constantly on call could speed to the scene, drop down and pick up the victims and be back at the trauma unit in a minimum of time. The long delays due to traffic congestion caused death, where helicopters without earth-bound delays saved lives. The cost was great but the commitment to life seemed to warrant the increased cost.

The medical director of an intensive care unit for high risk premature babies and neonatal emergencies which serves about a thousand newborns each year has worked out an arrangement with the Air National Guard for helicopter service. Here the costs are met by society and are spread through the tax burden. A few decades ago such costs were non-existent. Now they are part of the growing problem.

A friend who is a college professor spends time each week on a dialysis machine. He is able to stay alive and useful only because this expensive equipment is available. So much of modern medical practice is tied to sophisticated equipment of a mechanical nature that the cost factor becomes a constantly increasing part of medical intervention. If everyone who could benefit from such equipment had it to use the total cost of health care would increase considerably.

Computerized diagnosis and communication with data banks calls for sophisticated and expensive equipment, as does the use of X-ray diagnosis and radiation therapy. The more impersonal mechanical equipment medical practice employs, the more expensive health care tends to be. This too affects the emotional responses of patients.

The largest industry in the USA is the chemical business. Biomedical practice depends largely on the creations of the pharmaceutical laboratories, which are constantly at work to develop new methods for modifying body chemistry and interfering with the course of destructive viral influences. This form of external intervention adds to all the other costs mentioned so that health care becomes an even greater financial burden for a needy populace.

A major employer in most communities is the health care industry. Three shifts of hospital and nursing home personnel means that the ratio of paid workers to patients is about one to one. Specialized workers for complex equipment increases with the sophistication of the tools employed in the healing arts. No end is in sight.

The cost of education adds significantly to health care costs. The initial cost of premedical and medical education may be one hundred thousand dollars or more. Equipping an office may add fifty thousand more. High interest costs plus malpractice insurance can run into tens of thousands before the practitioner begins to realize anything for personal need. Continuing education adds even more expense. I work as a consultant for a medical publisher and know something of the prohibitive cost of medical books, which are highly specialized and used by a limited group of specialists.

All of these costs become part of the problem as we look towards the future. Biomedical practice tends to depend more and more on equipment, expanded staffs and heavy professional costs. The cost trend that now exists seems to indicate that traditional medical practice knows no other way to function. The cumulative burden can become so great that it grows intolerable and the biomedical approach to health care will destroy itself from within. Alternative approaches to this form of health care may be one of the ways of helping to prevent this form of self-destruction.

The threat of the mechanical is seen not only in the elaboration and glorification of machines. It also exists in the growing authority of the mechanical over the human. Futurists are concerned about the power of computers to assert mastery over life. If you have ever tried to correct a computer error you know how difficult it is. In just a few decades the computer has assumed power over us not imagined until recently.

One of the major challenges of the future has to do with the ability of the creators of the computer to reassert authority over their creation. Will we control the computer or will it control and master us? Aside from the military, in no field is this question more pertinent than in the field of biomedical practice where diagnosis and prognosis are increasingly entrusted to electronic equipment. The problem becomes most acute at the point where many important human considerations are not reducable to the formulas that can be fed into the machines. Much that is significantly human must then be ignored. The essentially human perceptions then may be slowly eliminated from consideration as the blatantly mechanical and materialistic aspects of being are enhanced. If human responses cannot be reduced to the statistical form that is amenable to the requirements of the computer, for all practical purposes they do not exist.

Mechanistic science has produced marvels of control in technical matters and electronics. If this skill can be used to aid humanity in the health care field, it could be a beneficial resource. But if the demands of technology supersede the needs of humans it is inevitable that the dehumanizing of medical practice will be carried a step further in the decades that lie ahead.

The explosion of knowledge makes specialization a necessity. At AMA headquarters in Chicago forty staff members are constantly at work scanning, analysing and checking out the ideas that come to them through the pages of the more than two thousand regularly published medical journals from all over the world. It is far from possible for a specialist to keep up with research in his own limited field. A stomatologist and a proctologist, dealing with different ends of the alimentary canal, are oriented about completely different types of research. In order to stay current with the specialization the physician focusses on a limited area of research and practice and in the very process reduces awareness of much else that is going on in the totality of medical research. But that is the only way the explosion of knowledge can be managed and as the practitioners know more and more about less and less the significance of the whole person may be reduced.

While some of the benefits of specialization are quite obvious, the tacit implications cannot be ignored. Students are expected to declare an area of specialization before leaving medical school. This provides the opportunity and incentive for further and more explicit training in the area of specialization. It is impossible to keep up with all areas of research and practice so the selection of a limited and limiting field for further exploration seems both reasonable and practical.

The implications of this procedure are that medical trainees will become more and more pre-occupied with one aspect of the patient's care and less and less concerned about the whole person. A basic question for the future seems to be: How can we preserve the benefits of specialized knowledge of the parts without losing the perspectives that are essentially related to the functioning of the total person? For the person is always more than the sum of the parts.

A specialist tends to be set apart as the recipient of special privileges and benefits. As a class they have the benefit of referrals so in effect the rest of the medical profession works for them. They can charge larger fees and be treated with deference. The granting of special status to those who specialize in parts tends to support a medical philosophy that moves away from a person as a person. By implication the general practitioner, who is more apt to be concerned about the total person, is reduced in status.

In contrast the ancillary forms of health care, osteopathy, naturopathy, chiropractic, etc., make a strong point of activating a total human response. They listen to the patient as well as talk with them. They encourage the patient to participate in the healing process. They work to create a partnership with the patient in restoration of health. The healer and the person being healed share responsibility as they work together to achieve health of body, mind and spirit.

Some deep human response resents being treated as less than human – a thing – an 'it' instead of a 'thou'. If specialization tends towards the impersonal it will be important to discover ways to reverse the trend. Dr Harry Lipscomb, a specialist in internal medicine, may be pointing the way towards a form of practice that brings together the benefits of specialization and the active resources resident in his patients.

Dr Lipscomb served as professor of internal medicine at Baylor Medical School. He was chosen to monitor the internal responses of astronauts in outer space. Before him on the television screens at NASA headquarters were the graphs of the various electronic devices attached to the bodies of the men in space. They showed the condition of skin, blood pressure, cardio-vascular response along with respiration and glandular reactions. In fact, sitting at his station in Houston he had a graphic picture of the near total response of the men in space.

Dr Lipscomb told me that when a crisis developed in space every body system of the astronauts was instantly activated. The monitors showed significant deviations from the normal in the body's response. Each system, in its own way, reacted to emotional stress. When the crisis was over the body functions returned to normal bounds.

Dr Lipscomb said that it would be difficult to return to his former mode of medical practice after participating in this dramatic demonstration of the total involvement of a person in crisis. He says that now he makes a specific effort to activate each patient as a partner in the healing process. For instance, when the patient comes for treatment, he does a complete workup on the patient and then shares his findings. In effect he says: this is all we have found out about you; several plausible treatment alternatives are open to us. Then after explaining them he asks the patient which makes the most sense from his or her point-of-view. This invites the patient to give emotional support to the healing process. Instead of being a passive and perhaps resistant observer, the patient is committed to a goal as an active partner. Dr Lipscomb says that he feels the results from this approach are positive and that the attitude of the patient hastens the processes of healing. He added that this form of active partnership also seems to effectively reduce the possibilities of a malpractice suit.

When patients have only a passive role and things go wrong they can resort only to legal processes to express their feelings. When they are active partners they have to share some of the responsibility. So from within medical practice, both as a form of self-defence and as a reasonable response to resources of the person that can be actively engaged, the benefits of specialization can be combined with the resources of the patient. Perhaps this is a clue to future forms of medical practice.

However, when a physician makes a patient a partner, there are certain changes in the relationship that must be faced. The physician must be willing to reduce authority and take a non-manipulative role. Part of the authority of the physician is claimed as a tacit right that goes with the implied contract that exists. In effect it says: you come to me because you recognize my special knowledge and skill; I have the right to exercise the authority that comes with the special knowledge and skill. I can take control of your life. I can give medicine, prescribe surgery and place you in medical re-straint in a hospital as a reasonable exercise of this authority.

Circumstances modify the use of authority. In a medical emergency the doctor's freedom to intervene may be greater than planning a long term programme of health care. When bleeding is profuse there is little question of a 'second opin-ion'. However, the general level of medical knowledge among lay people has increased and articles that are critical of medical practitioners tend to reduce authority and the power to manipulate. While the process may be moderate in tempo, it is quite obvious from decade to decade that the physician-patient relationship is being modified. Patients are withdrawing some of the authority previously granted and are increasingly resistant to manipulation. Such changes are part of a modification in health care practices and are shaping the mode of practice for the future.

The self-policing processes within the medical community have long taken a careful look at failures. When I was studying in classes of physicians who were reviewing treatment processes I was impressed by the persistence of the question, 'What happened to the patient?' With ruthless candour the therapeutic processes were examined with one thought uppermost, the end result as far as the patient was concerned. The within-house judgments were severe and devastating. Blame was directed where warranted and approval where deserved.

More recently the processes that assess competence have emerged from the protective climate of the professional community and are held up for public examination. Congressional committees hold hearings and reports indicate millions of unnecessary surgical interventions that cost four billion dollars and ten thousand lives. The Moss report further states that in three Massachusetts hospitals the rates of failure in open heart surgery were ten per cent, twenty-two per cent and forty-nine per cent. Persons living in the Boston area would naturally be interested in these statistics if they were in the market for open heart surgery.

Many of the failures that are the focus of criticism can be traced to misunderstandings of the differences that exist between emergency, clinical, terminal and general forms of practice. Short term relief from medical crises is quite different from long-term planning or ameliorative action. In short term activity the research in psychosomatics and psychogenics may not seem relevant. This does not imply that the research lacks validity. It merely indicates that it can be applied in varying degrees as situations warrant.

The insistence of pain calls for intervention to relieve the pain. But pain and responsibility are not unrelated. 'People have become unable to deal effectively with their suffering without professional intervention. But the experience of illness can serve as a nidus for a growing sense of personal responsibility for one's own health.'[1] To focus on relief of pain alone may in the long run impair a patient's ability to acquire the skill needed to be a more responsible person. Medical convenience and patient insistence are not enough to determine a total philosophy of medical practice.

Two things seem quite clear as we look towards the forms of health care in the future. In the first place we have from within medical practice itself signs of breakdown. Not only have the costs of biomedical care become excessive, but also its philosophical base tends to turn people into things rather than discovering the healing potential in each individual and using it to the extent of its possibility. Specialization as a side effect tends to fix the mechanical and impersonal into the system at the same time that it tends to enhance the power of the physician to take an authoritarian and manipulative stance. That means that some of the failures are built-in rather than self-correcting.

In the second place there is within medical research and practice a growing awareness of inadequacy. As two physicians put it, 'The scientific frame of reference, while revolutionizing our knowledge of people as organic entities, has failed to grasp fully our experience with patients and the spiritual and emotional forces which move them.'[2] The inclination for larger segments of society to take increased responsibility for their health can stimulate change within the biomedical community. How quickly and how effectively the medical establishment will respond to the demands for change both within and without may be determined by the pressures that are created by such ventures as this in which we are now engaged where the state of health care is looked at candidly, objectively and where suggestions for creative change are examined.

People grant authority and people can withdraw it when they feel it is no longer warranted. Tendencies in the direction of change are all about us. Some may be creative and useful.

Some may be unfortunate and destructive. As we look towards the release from self-imposed destructiveness through the larger perspectives of our maxi-system, we welcome a loyalty to something larger than our limited self-protectiveness. As we develop larger loyalties we move beyond our need to protect our smallness and our limited perspectives. We move towards a new freedom of mind and spirit that welcomes openness and mutually experiences candor for there is less to fear and more to be gained by our freedom to traverse new terrain of ideas and common hopes.

Human kind have long made a major investment of mind and emotion in the struggle to understand health. Many times they have confounded themselves by wanderings about in the compelled poverty of their many mini-systems. We have seen how people hobble themselves by their limited loyalties and cramped ways of thinking and acting. Now that we have seen the benefits of the larger perspectives that come with the larger systems approach, is there any reason for retreating to the old and inadequate ways of the past? We answer our own question by the way we think and act. We answer our question positively when we add religious conviction to our scientific discipline as we meld our efforts to create a new day in our understanding of health of body, mind and spirit. It may well be that we are closer to the time when that is not only a possibility but it may be a necessity as we seek to resolve the problems we have created for ourselves in biomedical practice and social insight. We stand at the threshhold of a new era. Will we take the opportunity or fail the future because we have failed to really understand the true nature of health?

Biomedical practice tends to operate with restraints that characterize a mini-system. Holistic health demands more of life as it tries to fulfill the goals of a maxi-system.

Conclusion: Towards the Twenty-First Century

The last decades of this century are now slipping away more rapidly than we are prepared to admit. Soon we will have terminated another millenium. What will we take with us into the new century and the new millenium? Will we be hobbled by limited scientific perspectives? Will we be able to build on the truth we have discovered to institute new ideas about health, holistic medicine and a concept of superhealthy people?

At the outset we know we have some large problems. We have been so immersed in a limiting scientific method that we have allowed it to become a philosophy. We have been so enamoured by technologies that we have elevated techniques to a way of life. The unique and wonderfully endowed human being has been discounted and the sources of inner strength have been ignored or abused. In the pages that lie behind us we have tried to explore what has happened to us, what it means in terms of health, what are the possibilities of building something more fruitful in the future, and what are the resources we possess for that building project. At best, our exploration has been limited and primarily suggestive. On the basis of what we have done, what can we say about where we are going and what can be done?

We know we have large resources. We know that science and research have provided us with material to be integrated such as has never existed in human history. Part of the problem is that we have so much that there appears to be no way of bringing it all together. Not long ago I spent a day with Leonard S. Cottrell, former dean of Cornell University and more recently a social scientist for the Russell Sage Foundation. He was asked to lay aside all other activities and give two years of his life to the task of reorganizing and co-ordinating the total scientific and research projects that were in any way subsidized by the federal government. In a paragraph it is impossible to do justice to the monumental work Dr Cottrell did in trying to bring order out of chaos and set a course for the future in science and research. But some of his insights can be useful for us in suggesting some of the course of the future. We are now faced with a glut of knowledge and information that cannot be easily organized because there is no unifying language and there is no unifying philosophy that can amalgamate our vast reservoir of knowledge and information. As I was leaving after hours of fruitful conversation he handed me two papers he had written. One was a sophisticated and complicated discussion of a formula for bringing together the voluminous research sponsored by our government. The other was a very personal paper about the religious experience he had as he looked back over a long and fruitful life working on the frontiers of the personality and social sciences for nearly half a century. The things that were ultimately important for him did not deal with quantity as much as quality, with measurement as much as meaning, with research as much as a religious organization of life and its purpose. The ancient questions persist. The current answers may merely confuse and distort unless the language of meaning can be rediscovered and the processes of revelation can be used to bring together in purpose and meaning what might be otherwise flung further apart by the centrifugal impulse of scientific research, each discipline going its own way farther and farther into the unknown without markers to aid in finding the way back.

There was a time when human experience could be organized geographically but modern travel has obliterated our boundaries for all practical purposes though we go on acting as if we believe in them. Cities illustrate this phenomenon. Lewis Mumford writes: 'The city is a special receptacle for storing and transmitting messages. The development of symbolic methods of storage immensely increased the capacity of the city as a container; it not only held together a larger body but it maintained and transmitted a larger portion of their lives than individual human memories could transmit by word of mouth.' As cities became centres for technology they tended to serve as unifiers of life. Often this sense of unity was misleading. The Roman Catholic Church which has had a long tradition of trying to bring together disparate elements of society, has tried to find a common denominator for faith and knowledge to reconcile science and technology with religion. One prelate of the church has said: 'The church today finds herself face to face with a new kind of Koine, that is, a universal way of thinking and speaking. This Koine is a product of progress in technology which is valid across all frontiers and iron curtains.' Jean Cardinal Danielou said, 'Nothing is more biblical than technology.' To glorify technology as if it were the great deliverer may well start us off on a quest for security where it does not exist. The technology that ignores the boundaries of space and time also creates the devices that can ignore boundaries and people and the cities in which they live. Technology may be a useful slave but an unpredictable master.

Lewis Mumford looks more realistically at the conflict between the tyranny of techniques and the hegemony of humanity when he writes in *The Myth of the Machine*:

The present analysis of techniques and human development rests on belief in the imperative need for reconciling and fusing together the subjective and the objective aspects of human experience, by a methodology that will ultimately embrace both. This can come about, not by dismissing either religion or science, but first by detaching them from the obsolete ideological matrix that has distorted their respective developments and limited their field of interaction. Man's marvellous achievements in projecting his subjective impulses into institutional forms, aesthetic symbols, mechanical organizations, and architectural structures have been vastly augmented by the orderly co-operative methods that science has exemplified and universalized. But at the same time, to reduce acceptable subjectivity to the ideal level of a computer would only sever rationality and order from their deepest sources in the organism. If we are to save technology itself from the aberrations of its present leaders and putative gods, we must, in both our thinking and our acting, come back to the human centre: for it is there that all significant transformations begin and germinate.[1]

Biomedical practice that increasingly depends on mechanical devices, electronic techniques and computers may wander away from the human centre and lose sight of its ultimate purpose in bringing health to the people it serves. Like the Pentagon of Power that may destroy humankind in order to save it, the non-rational philosophical base that develops when we move away from the human centre may gain ascendency and all else move into decline.

Our approach to the twenty-first century will undoubtedly rest on an expanded sense of responsibility. Responsibility is basically an answer to circumstance. It is a response to life in terms of its ultimate meaning. As we conclude our brief survey of the state of health care as we enter a new century we cannot ignore the response we make to the history upon which we must build. This calls for an awareness of personal, social, scientific and spiritual forms of responsibility.

We have seen the great upsurge of personal responsibility for types of health care. This tends to express itself in more and

131

more individualized concerns for diet and exercise of body, mind and spirit. This tendency towards organized self-interest may lead towards conceiving health as an end in itself. This preoccupation of health for health's sake may well play into the hands of those who would make all health problems a matter of limited self-interest and thus restrain those who would face the social dimension of environmental forces and collective interest in creating an increasingly healthful, disease-free climate for life.

Those who take their health into their own hands may be turning their backs on a resource that they may desperately need. In another context it has been pointed out that a person who is determined to be his own lawyer may have a fool for a client. A person who carries health care to an exclusion of medical resources may find that self-diagnosis is not only expensive, but can produce many complications. Doctors may err in diagnosis but there is no doubt that they have a broader base for understanding what is going on physically than those who have little or no background in the precise sciences involved. The alternatives are not completely spelled out in a choice between meditation and medication. The either-or may be improved by a both-and.

In a world of specialists the practice of self-diagnosis may be even more unacceptable. A young woman, married four years, and in excellent health, began to have dizzy spells. Because she felt she knew more about herself than anyone else she decided her eyes needed testing. The eye specialist told her her eyes were perfect and made an appropriate charge. Not to be defeated she decided the next possibility was her heart so she went to a cardiologist who found her heart was in excellent condition and he made an appropriate charge. In increasing desperation she thought it might be in her head so she went to a psychiatrist who found her to be psychologically sound and made an appropriate charge. After all this she blurted it out to her husband who suggested their family

132

physician. His examination completed he said, 'Eat good food, get plenty of rest and in eight months or so your problems will be resolved with a bundle of joy.' Most people have insufficient experience to practice a skilled profession on their own. The wisdom of sound personal interest in health care can be supplemented by a wise use of the medical resources available.

Social responsibility goes hand in hand with personal health care. Holistic health perceptions are apt to be understood and practiced by a privileged segment of society and it would be unwise to exclude the rest of society from the benefits of socially concerned health care. What would be especially true of infants, children and the aged, could also be true for the underprivileged.

The impact of society on the quality of life has a statistical base. The death rate among children in the year 1900 in the USA was fifty-six per cent of the total death count in the country. Now the number of child deaths is less than six per cent. This major demographic shift is credited to the social control of infectious disease. Life expectancy during the same period has moved from forty-six to seventy-two years of age. This reflects the major change in the management of childhood and other infectious disease. Yet the life expectancy of men over sixty has increased only two per cent during the same time. The life expectancy of Blacks still lags behind Whites. 'Nor has modern medicine devised many successful modes of dealing with chronic diseases, which seem to have unnecessarily high rates of morbidity and mortality.'[2]

If an active interest in holistic health is used to divert attention and research activity away from specific social needs in health care, sooner or later we will all be the losers. So it is not a matter of personal or social responsibility that faces us in the future, but rather the matter of exploring the best ways of combining personal and social interest to meet the needs of the present that are clearly being projected into the future.

133

In addition to all that can be done to develop patterns of personal concern and life-styles affecting health, the needs of society are better systems for providing health research, health insurance and health care.

Scientific responsibility is also called for. This is important in both research and health care delivery systems. Large amounts of government, private and public funds have been made available for cancer research. This has been centred on traditional forms of biomedical exploration. Even though significant results have been gained in psychotherapeutic intervention and holistic approaches to the prevention and treatment of cancer, funds for this type of research have been largely non-existent. Vested interest in research has amplified the basic assumptions of a philosophy that is cell-centred rather than person-centred so that in this research the human centre is largely ignored. My family has been deeply engrossed in cancer research for sixty years, so I have had a chance to observe how research programmes have developed. Having served as a consultant for the National Cancer Institute as well as having received an award from the American Cancer Society I have been actively interested in the human side of the cancer problem. If as much money were made available for research in the psychogenic and immunological aspects of cancer development and treatment as is spent on chemotherapy, radiation chemistry and surgical intervention, I would feel that we would be farther ahead in our control of this baffling cluster of cellular behaviour manifestations. If the future is to be well served the vested interests of individuals and institutions in traditional forms of research will need to be re-examined from the base of broader human interests and the psychodynamics that have such significant etiological correlations.

The results of intensive research over more than half a century have produced limited results and the needs of the future call for a more audacious approach to the human centre that creates the metaphoric language that tells much about both the person and the society. New skills in studying this language can open doors of research and treatment that may hasten the triumph over malignant responses of the living organism in the next century. Will medical science move beyond the laboratory to learn the language of the body and pay attention to what it is saying about both people and the society in which they live?

Probably basic changes in personal, social and scientific goals can come only when there is a supportive spiritual climate. Spirituality is always personal. The only place where it can develop is within individuals. There are institutions that can stimulate an interest in the development of the human spirit but there are no spiritual institutions as such. There are philosophies of life that can provide the launching pad for daring concepts of the human spirit and its potential but there are no spiritual philosophies except as people spiritualize them. Too often we have tried to provide spiritual incentives for life from the outside when they can only be generated from within by the nurturing and disciplining of the power of human consciousness. That which is made in the image of God can only achieve its potential when it is done through active relationship between the human spirit and the cosmic spirit. Here the bonding that begins at the physical level in the trust of the infant can achieve another and more significant level of social bonding in adolescence and be fulfilled in the mating or parental bond in adulthood, and achieve its highest form of expression in the cosmic bond that brings all of life into a relationship of creature and creator, the inner self and the beyond self, the human being and the cosmic being.

Research in the personality sciences now makes it possible for us to appreciate the deeper meaning of the New Testament revelation. We are called upon to develop the inner possibilities of our disciplined consciousness to undergird holistic concepts of health through personal responsibility, social responsibility, scientific responsibility and spiritual responsibility. If the future is going to move beyond 'more of the same' to bold new ventures into the possibilities of more healthful persons and a deeply concerned society, it will be through motivation that grows out of a meaning for life that transcends the material, physical and artifical to release the extra-sensory, transpersonal and spiritual to fulfil the accumulated personal and social potential of the human spirit, set free from enslaving mini-systems and fulfilled through the disciplined power of consciousness. Then the God within will activate the power within that will manifest itself in newness of life.

If there is anything we have learned from our encounter with the AIDS phenomenon it is that immediate action is of the essence. What was undiscovered and unknown in medical practice a few years ago is now at the centre of our concerns. Without going into the dynamics of the disease we are very much aware of the fact that it has a destructive power of its own that can spread anxiety and human misery. It rivals the nuclear threat as a possible final catastrophe for the human race. The ability to establish a measure of control over its deadly power is measured in years not in centuries. The scenario for the future of the race faces us with alternatives that do not allow time for temporizing and makeshift ways of doing things. We cannot win the battle by partial actions or delaying tactics. We are faced with the need for major changes in people and societies, behaviour patterns and established values.

We have no clearly established way of moving against the threat if we try to meet it with our outworn ideas of ethical standards and moral precepts. We need not only completely new ways of looking at our human crisis but a determination to make the major changes in commitment and action that are adequate to the human crisis that faces humankind. This calls for changes so complete that our ideas of national sovereignty and social controls will have to be adjusted to their inadequacy for the task.

We are led to believe that nearly half of the physicians in the USA – and this is probably true of the whole Western world – do not want anything to do with AIDS patients. That gives us an idea of how much change is needed in the professional group most involved. The fear and anxiety prevalent will first have to be dealt with. Only then and in the deeper levels of society will the courage be developed to make major changes in attitude and practice.

Perhaps the stimulus of a crisis such as the AIDS epidemic can give will hasten some of the activity that has been impeded by small loyalties and unwillingness to venture beyond the bounds set by a mini-system. At one time happiness was considered to be freedom from sin and a mini-system was created to absolve people from their sins. Now it is freedom from disease and the mini-system of biomedical philosophy and practice works to bring that form of happiness to humankind.

Perhaps we are at a turning point in history. We face forces that are destructive in massive form. But we also are the first generation in human history endowed with the psychology of consciousness and the physics of energy-processes that make it possible for us to understand the revelation of the nature of God and the power within that Jesus revealed through his life and teaching. The question is whether we will accept the challenge of these times of great possibility, or retreat in fear back to the old days of thinking and feeling? What happens in these years that lead us into the twenty-first century will be our answer.

Notes

1. From Fractions to Wholes

1. *The New Illustrated Medical Encyclopaedia* ed. Robert E. Rothenberg, vol. 4, Abradale Press, NY 1959.

2. See, for instance, Lawrence LeShan and Edgar N. Jackson, *How to Meditate*, Evans, NY 1977

3. Leonard Cottrell, *Identity and Interpersonal Competence*, University of Chicago Press 1955.

4. Sally Guttmacher, 'Whole in Body, Mind and Spirit' in *The Hastings Center Report*, vol. 9, no. 2, April 1979, p. 17.

5. Ibid.

2. Spiritual Bases of the Meld

1. Alexis Carrel, *The Voyage to Lourdes*, Harper & Row, NY 1950.

2. George Santyana, *Skepticism and Animal Faith*, Constable 1923.

3. Lawrence LeShan, *The Medium, the Mystic and the Physicist*, Viking Press, NY 1975.

4. Robert Laidlaw, *From Wainwright House Reports*, Fifth Spiritual Healing Seminar, Rye, NY 1956.

5. George Devereaux, *Psychoanalysis and the Occult*, International University Press 1970; Shafica Karagula, *Breakthrough to Creativity*, De Vorss, Los Angeles 1968.

6. Lawrence LeShan, op. cit.

3. A Systems Approach

1. Harry Rudin, Professor of History at Yale University, in a public lecture.

2. Edgar Douglas Adrian, Master of Trinity, Cambridge, has done important research on brain waves and the nervous system, and was awarded a Nobel Prize for Medicine for work on the function of neurons; Sir John Eccles, a New Zealand neurosurgeon, has done research on the brain and its function, the mind and its meaning.

3. American Foundation, *Medical Research: A Midcentury Survey*, Little Brown, Boston 1955, vol. 2, pp. 4f.

4. Ervin Laszlo, *A Systems View of the World*, Blackwell 1972, pp. 23, 41.

5. Edmund Pellegrino, 'Philosophy of Medicine: Problematic and Potential' in *The Journal of Medicine and Philosophy*, vol. 1, no. 1, March 1976, p. 7.

6. Ibid., p. 5.

7. T. Boyce and M. Michael, 'Nine Assumptions of Western Medicine' in *Man and Medicine*, vol. 1, no. 4, Summer 1976, pp. 317ff.

8. Jerome Frank, article in *Archives of Neurology and Psychiatry*, vol. 77, pp. 283–99.

9. Ibid.

10. David Bakan, *Disease, Pain and Sacrifice*, University of Chicago Press 1968, p. 29.

11. James J. Lynch, *The Broken Heart*, Basic Books, NY 1977, pp. 87ff.

12. Ibid.

4. Using Inner Resources

1. Lawrence LeShan and Edgar N. Jackson, *How to Meditate*, 'Afterword – The Three Force Fields', Evans, NY 1977.

2. Lawrence LeShan, *Alternative Realities*, Evans, NY 1976.

3. J. Jaynes, *The Origin of Consciousness*, Houghton Mifflin, NY 1976, p. 446.

4. M. Eliade, *Myth and Reality*, Harper Colophon Books, NY 1963; D. Malinowski, *The Death of the Gods*, Modern Library, NY 1929.

5. J. Campbell, *The Mythic Image*, The Bollinger Series, Princeton University Press 1974.

5. Self Organizing Self

1. The concept of prenatal self-image or body-image has long been surmised by scriptural references (eg. Ps. 22.9; 149.13). Gary Benfield, Director of the premature birth trauma unit of Akron Children's Hospital, works on that premise with massage of babies two or three months short of term. Nandor Fodor wrote a book on *The New Interpretation of Dreams* which assumes prenatal experience is reflected in dream content. Carl Jung was sure that archetypal and preconscious material came from prenatal development. More recently, LeBoyer bases a mode of infant care on relating body experience with the experience following birth. Bruner, in *The First Relationship*, builds

on the prenatal development, and William Johnston in *The Mirror Mind* (Harper 1981), in a section on 'From the Womb to the Tomb', gives added references to this ancient and contemporary assumption.

2. James J. Lynch, 'The Psychological Impact of Early Loss', *The Broken Heart*, Basic Books, NY 1977, pp. 75–79.

3. Jacob Needleman, *A Sense of the Cosmos*, Doubleday 1975, p. 47.

4. Jerome F. Frederick, 'Possible Failure of Immunosurveillance System' in *Grief and Cancer*, College of Physicians and Surgeons Symposium on Acute Grief, Columbia University, NY 1980.

6. Mysticism

1. Herman Hesse, *The Journey to the East*, Panther 1973.

2. Alan Watts, *The Spirit of Zen*, John Murray 1948, pp. 45ff.

3. Mary Baker Eddy, *Science and Health*, first published 1875 and reissued many times by the Christian Science publishing house in Boston.

4. Albert Abrams, *New Concepts in Diagnosis and Treatment*, Philopolis Press, San Francisco 1916.

5. For Freud's conflict with materialistic philosophy see his *The Future of Illusion*, Hogarth Press 1962 and *Moses and Monotheism*, Hogarth Press 1951; both also included in *Collected Papers*, 5 vols, Hogarth Press 1956–57.

6. Edwin Burtt, *The Metaphysical Foundations of Modern Physical Science*, Doubleday 1954.

7. Albert Einstein, *Cosmic Religion*, Covici Friede, NY 1931.

8. Max Planck, *Scientific Autobiography*, Philosophical Library, NY 1949, last page.

9. Henry Margenau, in personal correspondence with me.

10. Pierre Teilhard de Chardin, *Science and Christ*, Harper & Row, NY 1965 and Collins, London 1968.

7. Learning from Historical Perspectives

1. T. Boyce and M. Michael, 'Nine Assumptions of Western Medicine' in *Man and Medicine*, vol. 1, no. 4, Summer 1976, pp. 317ff.

2. Ibid., p. 317.

8. A Broadening Awareness

1. T. Boyce and M. Michael, 'Nine Assumptions of Western Medicine' in *Man and Medicine*, vol. 1, no. 4, Summer 1976, p. 311–12.

2. W. Cannon, *Bodily Changes in Pain, Hunger, Fear and Rage*, Appleton, NY 1929.

3. W. Cannon, *The Wisdom of the Body*, Norton, NY 1932.

4. H. F. Dunbar, *Emotions and Bodily Change*, Columbia University Press 1935.

5. *The New Illustrated Medical Encyclopaedia* ed. Robert E. Rothenberg, Abradale Press, NY 1959.

6. A glossary of these terms may be helpful in their proper use. *Placebo response* refers to the change produced in a patient when an inert substance is used in place of the specific medication usually prescribed. The landmark work of Jerome Frank in this field has been supplemented more recently by the work of William Lamers with the creating of peptides such as endorphine and enkephaline. A combination of suggestion, expectancy, personality characteristics of the patient and the authority of the person administering the placebo appear to be significant contributors to the process.

Homeostasis is the term used to describe the chemical balance within the body when it is functioning within the normal range of healthful body function.

Intropsychic balance is the term that describes a state of coping skills as the person encounters emotional stress and wisely manages it. Karl Menninger in his book *The Vital Balance* elaborates on this term and its meaning.

Psychosomatic is the term that describes the state of constant inter-relationship between the physical body and the non-physical factors that are perpetually impinging on the body. The term describes a relationship between the psyche and soma in Greek terminology and does not define a specific cause-effect process.

Psychogenic, in contrast, makes specific the genesis or causative factor in the psyche with the assumption of its effect upon the body. All psychogenic illness is psychosomatic but not all psychogenic manifestations are psychosomatic because there are other causative influences at work in life such as heredity, environment, ageing and accidents as well as attitudes.

7. Dr L. E. Hinkle and Dr H. G. Wolff, paper read at the American Medical Association Convention in 1957 and reprinted in *The Creative Power of the Mind*, Prentice Hall, NJ 1957, p. 203.

8. 'Stress Preceded Onset of Disease' in *Brain/Mind*, 2(15), 1977.

9. Erich Lindemann, article in *Journal of Psychiatry*, CI 1944, p. 147.

10. E. Weiss and S. English, 'Emotional Factors in Bronchial Asthma', *Psychosomatic Medicine*, Saunders, Philadelphia 1943, pp. 420f.; F. Alexander, 'Emotional Factors in Respiratory Disturbance', *Psychosomatic Medicine*, Norton 1950, pp. 132–42; H. F. Dun-

bar, 'Asthma', *Your Child's Mind and Body*, Random House, NY 1949, pp. 189–94.

11. J. F. Frederick, 'The Transmission of Malignant Diseases' in *The Dodge Magazine*, January 1975.

12. F. Dunbar, *Emotions and Bodily Changes*, Columbia University Press, NY 1954, pp. 170f.

13. Ibid., p. 541.

14. Lawrence LeShan, *You Can Fight for Your Life*, Evans, NY 1977.

15. J. Salk, 'Holistic Health Approach Inevitable in "Epoch B"' in *Brain/Mind*, 1977, 2.

16. Roy Menninger, *'Quo Vadis*, Medicine?' in *Brain/Mind*, 1977, 1(1).

9. New Partnerships

1. Ervin Laszlo, *A Systems View of the World*, Blackwell 1972.

2. In the long (4 years) and acrimonious discourse among Leibnitz, Arnauld and Count Hessen-Rheinfels which centred on conflicts between Lutherans and Catholic theologians, the role of Leibnitz was significant. In dealing with tertiary abstractions which are central to most theological debates Leibnitz pointed out that personal involvement was central, and that disputants were usually right when they spoke out of their own experience and belief but that was insufficient evidence to disqualify the insight of those who had different experience and belief. The lengthy exchange of correspondence is found in G. Leibnitz, *Discourse on Metaphysics: Correspondence with Arnauld and Monadology*, Open Court Publishing Company, Chicago 1931.

3. Definition of 'denial' in the *Psychiatric Dictionary*, OUP 1970.

4. Jerome F. Frederick, 'Epstein-Barr: Possible Failure of Immuno-surveillance System' in *The Dodge Magazine*, March and June 1976.

10. New Practices

1. 'Who Should Pay for Smokers' Medical Care?' in *The Hastings Center Report*, November 1974, pp. 8ff.

2. James A. Knight, *The Medical Student: Doctor in the Making*, Appleton-Century Crofts, NY 1973, p. 12.

3. See my *Coping with the Crises in Your Life*, Aronson, Ny 1980.

4. Viktor Frankl, *The Doctor and the Soul*, Alfred Knopf 1955.

5. *Catastrophic Illness: Impact on Families, Challenge to the Professions*, Cancer Care Inc., NY 1966, pp. 26–37.

11. New Research and New Skills

1. L. E. Abt and S. L. Weissman, *Acting Out*, Grune & Stratton, NY 1965.

2. Alvin Toffler, *Future Shock*, Random House, NY 1970.

3. Frederick LeBoyer, *Childbirth Without Violence*, Alfred Knopf, NY 1978 and *Loving Hands*, Knopf 1976, present his ideas with numerous illustrations.

4. Peterim A. Sorokin, *Altruistic Love*, Beacon Press, Boston 1959, pp. vf., 9, 23, 94f., 184.

5. Alexis Carrel, *Man, the Unknown*, Harper & Row, NY 1935, pp. 122f.

6. R. M. Bucke, *Cosmic Consciousness*, E. P. Dutton, NY 1968.

7. Glen Clark, *George Washington Carver, The Man Who Talked to Plants*, privately published pamphlet.

8. Albert Einstein, *Cosmic Religion*, Covici Friede, NY 1931, pp. 52ff.

12. The Need to Accelerate

1. T. Boyce and M. Michael, 'Nine Assumptions of Western Medicine' in *Man and Medicine*, vol. 1, no. 4, Summer 1976, p. 314.

2. Ibid., p. 317; see also A. Koestler, *The Ghost in the Machine*. Regenery, Chicago 1967, *Beyond Reductionism*, Beacon Press, Boston 1969, *The Roots of Coincidence* Vintage, NY 1972; M. Polanyi, *Personal Knowledge*, Routledge & Kegan Paul 1962; R. Poole, *Towards Deep Subjectivity*, Harper & Row, NY 1972.

Conclusion: Towards the Twenty-First Century

1. Lewis Mumford, *The Myth of the Machine*, Harcourt Brace Jovanovich, NY 1979, p. 420.

2. Sally Guttmacher, 'Whole in Body, Mind and Spirit' in *The Hastings Center Report*, vol. 9, no. 2, April 1979, p. 15.

For Further Reading

1. Books by doctors of medicine which start with a biomedical perception and move in various directions:

Richard Almond, *The Healing Community*, Aronson, NY 1974

Rebecca Beard, *Everyman's Search*, Arthur James 1962

Alexis Carrel, *Man, the Unkonwn*, Harper & Row, NY 1950

René Dubos, *Mirage of Health*, Doubleday Anchor Books, NY 1961

Flanders Dunbar, *Emotions and Bodily Changes*, Columbia University Press, NY 1956

B. J. Ficarra, *A Psychosomatic Approach to Surgery*, Froken Press, NY 1951

Jerome Frank, *Persuasion and Healing*, John Hopkins Press, Baltimore 1961

Viktor Frankl, *The Doctor and the Soul*, Alfred Knopf, NY 1953

Shafica Karagula, *Breakthrough to Creativity*, De Vorss, Los Angeles 1957

R. D. Laing, *Self and Others*, Pantheon Books, NY 1969

Henry Margenau, *The Miracle of Existence*, New Science Library, Boston 1987

Hans Selye, *The Stress of Life*, McGraw Hill, NY 1956

A. T. W. Simeons, *Man's Presumptuous Brain*, E. P. Dutton, NY 1961

E. F. Winkler, *Man, the Bridge Between Two Worlds*, Harper & Row, NY 1960

Worcester, McComb and Coreat, *Religion and Science*, Moffat, Yard and Co., NY 1908

2. Books written from a scientific and philosophical understanding of human beings and their natures

Albert Einstein, *Cosmic Religion*, Covici Freide, NY 1931
R. H. Kiernan, *General Smuts*, Harrap 1943
A. Koestler and J. Smythies, *Beyond Reductionism*, Beacon Press, Boston 1969
Ervin Laszlo, *A Systems View of the World*, Blackwell 1972
Lawrence LeShan, *You Can Fight for Your Life*, Evans, NY 1977
Catherine Lyons, *Organ Transplants: The Moral Issues*. Westminster Press, Philadelphia and SCM Press, London 1970
M. A. H. Melinsky (ed.), *Religion and Medicine Vols 1 & 2*, SCM Press, London 1970, 1973
D. W. Millard (ed.), *Religion and Medicine Vol. 3*, SCM Press, London 1976
Harold K. Schilling, *Science and Religion*, Scribners, NY 1962

3. Books written from a variety of more practical perspectives

William Dampier-Whetham, *A History of Science*, Macmillan, NY 1931
H. E. Fosdick, *On Being a Real Person*, Harper, NY and SCM Press, London 1943
Alister Hardy, *The Spiritual Nature of Man*, OUP 1979
Rosalind Heywood, *ESP: A Personal Memoir*, E. P. Dutton, NY 1964
Ashley Montagu, *Touching*, Columbia University Press 1971
Joseph Needham (ed.), *Science, Religion and Reality*, George Braziller, NY 1955
W. L. Northbridge, *Disorders of the Emotional and Spiritual Life*, Channel Press, Great Neck, NY 1961
Bertrand Russell, *The Impact of Science on Society*, Simon and Schuster, NY 1953
Edmond Sinnott, *Two Roads to Truth*, Viking Press, NY 1953

4. Journals and periodicals

The Hastings Center Report, 360 Broadway, Hastings-on-the-Hudson, NY 10706

Brain/Mind, PO Box 42211, Los Angeles, Cal. 90042

Man and Medicine, Columbia University of Physicians and Surgeons, 630 West 168th Street, NY 10032

The Menninger Bulletin, Topeka, Kansas

The Dodge Magazine published in Cambridge, Mass. for the Dodge Chemical Laboratory, Bronx, NY